Blockmate

Arunangshu Chakraborty
Editor

Blockmate

A Practical Guide for Ultrasound Guided Regional Anaesthesia

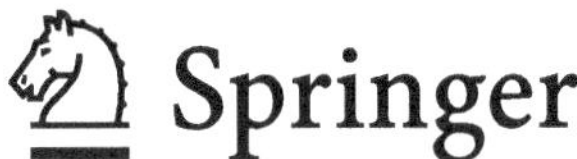

Editor
Arunangshu Chakraborty
Department of Anaesthesia, CC and Pain
Tata Medical Center
Kolkata
India

ISBN 978-981-15-9204-1 ISBN 978-981-15-9202-7 (eBook)
https://doi.org/10.1007/978-981-15-9202-7

This Springer imprint is published by the registered company Springer Nature Singapore Pte Ltd.
The registered company address is: 152 Beach Road, #21-01/04 Gateway East, Singapore 189721, Singapore

This work is dedicated to our parents who always saw our potential and nurtured our dreams.

We convey special thanks to our families who sacrificed their time and allowed us to complete this task, which sometimes seemed like never ending.

Above all, we thank God almighty without whose permission nothing happens in this world.

Preface

Regional anaesthesia has seen a resurgence of interest among anaesthesiologists in the recent past. The block techniques, obscure and unsure, hitherto have found validation in the clear imagery of ultrasound. Ultrasound-guided regional anaesthesia (USRA) over the last decade has become the standard of care and thereby a valuable skill in the repertoire of the anaesthesiologist. While the techniques are many and interesting, we found that there is a dearth of handy textbooks that the anaesthesiology resident or practitioner can carry in his pocket and use in the operating room for ready reference. The chapters in this book are brief, illustrative and problem oriented, ideal for the trainee or practitioner who is about to start his journey of regional anaesthesia practice. We have covered almost all the blocks in practice in anatomical order and given a brief introduction to the basics of ultrasound for ease of apprehension. The book also contains a chapter on safety and ergonomics of USRA, which is very important for the trainee, and a chapter on recent and upcoming advances in the field. While we will be bringing in new editions as the field of regional anaesthesia gets updated, we will appreciate the feedback from our readers. Please do write to us and let us know what you liked or disliked about our book and what more do you want from this book in the future editions.

Kolkata, India — Arunangshu Chakraborty

Acknowledgement

I thankfully acknowledge the invaluable contribution of Dr. Ashokka Balakrishnan, MD, DNB, FANZCA, MHPE EDRA, without whose help this book would not have seen the light of the day. He has been a one-point solution for all the hurdles that I faced with the book. From connecting with contributing authors to getting his residents to draw the required diagrams, he has helped me overcome all the stumbling blocks of "blockmate". I thank Dr. Shri Vidya for finding out time to help us with the diagrams. I thank our colleagues who helped us to collect the images and the volunteers and patients who gave their kind permission for using their images for this book. Lastly, I thank all my co-authors for their valuable contributions.

Contents

About the Editor

Arunangshu Chakraborty, MBBS, MD graduated from Nil Ratan Sircar Medical College, Kolkata; obtained postgraduate qualification in anaesthesiology from Moti Lal Nehru Medical College, Allahabad; and pursued clinical fellowship at National University Hospital, Singapore. He is a consultant anaesthesiologist at Tata Medical Center, Kolkata, India, which is a tertiary level oncology centre. His areas of interest include regional anaesthesia, onco-anaesthesia and medical ultrasound. He has several peer-reviewed international publications and delivered many oral presentations in national and international level meetings. He has edited and authored a textbook on regional anaesthesia. He is an executive committee member of the Academy of Regional Anaesthesia, India, and reviewer of many international peer-reviewed medical journals.

1 Basics of Ultrasound Guided Regional Anaesthesia

Arunangshu Chakraborty and Ipsita Chattopadhyay

1.1 Basics of Ultrasound: Physics and Physiology

Sound waves are waves of compression and rarefaction in a medium such as air. For the propagation of sound, the most important factors are its frequency, wavelength and the qualities of the medium it travels through.

Only a part of the sound waves present in nature is audible to human ears, which is known as the *hearing range*. Human hearing range is between 20 and 20,000 Hz, although individual capabilities may vary. Any sound which has a frequency lower than 20 Hz is not audible to most humans and known as infrasound. On the other hand, the sound of frequency greater than 20,000 Hz is also inaudible to human ears and known as *ultrasound*. In the animal kingdom animals such as elephants can generate and hear the infrasound that allows them to communicate over a long distance, whereas bats and dolphins can generate and receive ultrasound which endows them survival edge in navigation and spatial orientation.

Ultrasound has steadily gained importance and popularity in medical imaging since its introduction in the early 1960s [1]. It has evolved rapidly through scientific discoveries and advancements in computing. When ultrasound was used for the first time in regional anaesthesia in the 1990s, the ultrasound output was a chart of dots. Now it provides real-time image which is easily relatable to the anatomy. Ultrasound is safer compared to ionising radiations and it is portable. The side effects of clinical ultrasound are negligible. Use of ultrasound by anaesthesiologists for the purpose of interventions such as vascular cannulations and regional anaesthesia have made those techniques safer and more reliable compared to the landmark-based techniques [2, 3].

A. Chakraborty (✉)
Department of Anaesthesia, CC and Pain, Tata Medical Center, Kolkata, India

I. Chattopadhyay
Department of Pain Medicine, R.G. Kar Medical College and Hospital, Kolkata, India

A. Chakraborty (ed.), *Blockmate*, https://doi.org/10.1007/978-981-15-9202-7_1

1.2 Mechanism of Action

Ultrasound is created by the piezoelectric effect (PE) converting electrical energy into mechanical vibrations (Fig. 1.1). The word piezo is derived from the Greek word 'piezein', meaning 'to press'. It was discovered by Pierre Curie in 1880 in quartz crystals.

When a varying voltage is applied, the PE material starts to vibrate, with the frequency of the voltage determining the frequency of the sound waves produced. When placed in contact with skin via an 'acoustic coupling' jelly, the 'transducer' (commonly called 'probe') transmits and receives the ultrasound beam.

The pulse wave that is generated at the transducer is transmitted into the body of the subject, reflected off the tissue interface and returned to the transducer again. These returning ultrasound waves cause the PE elements to vibrate within the transducer which causes a voltage to be generated. Thus, the same crystals are used to send and receive ultrasound waves. An image is created out of the returning signal.

With advancements in digital signal processing and software tools, the ultrasound image has evolved from a greyscale chart to a 3D image over the last four decades.

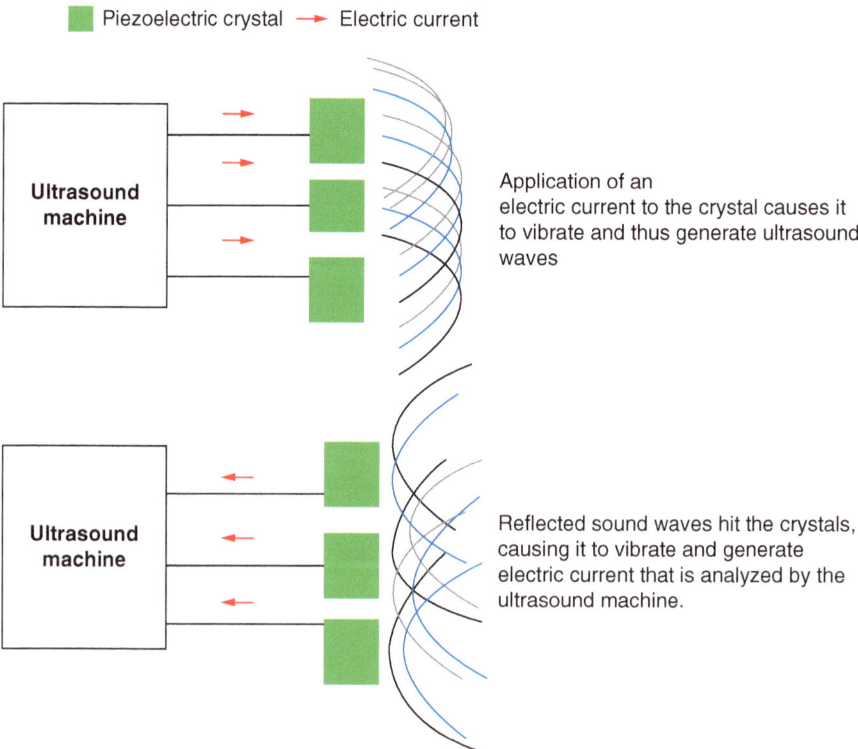

Fig. 1.1 Ultrasound created by piezoelectric effect converting electrical energy into mechanical vibrations

1.3 Key Concepts [4–6]

1. *Acoustic velocity (c)* is the speed at which sound waves travel through a medium. It is directly proportional to the density and stiffness of the medium.
   - The velocity is fastest in solids and slowest in air.

   The average speed of propagation of ultrasound in body tissue is about 1540 m/s.

2. *Acoustic Impedance* is the product of sound velocity and tissue density. The difference in acoustic impedance between two tissues influences the amplitude of the returning echo.
3. *Resolution* is the ability to distinguish between two structures that are positioned close to each other.

   Resolution depends on the frequency of ultrasound. Wavelength of the ultrasound beam is inversely proportional to the frequency. Smaller the wavelength, the better is the resolution. Thus, higher frequency gives better resolution.

   Resolution can be classified as spatial and temporal.

Spatial Resolution It is the ability of ultrasound to distinguish between two objects lying side by side. It can be of two types, axial and lateral.

- *Axial Resolution*: This is the ability to separately discern two structures lying along the ultrasound beam axis as separate and distinct. Affected by the frequency of the beam (Fig. 1.2). For example, when an abdominal wall is imaged, the ultrasound beam traverses the skin, subcutaneous tissue, the abdominal wall muscles with their fasciae, peritoneum and abdominal contents depending on the depth setting. A good resolution allows to distinguish between each of these structures separately.

- *Lateral Resolution*: It is the ability to distinguish between structures lying perpendicular to the beam axis, i.e. structures lying side by side. It is affected by the beam width (Fig. 1.3). For example, when the ultrasound scan is done for an

Fig. 1.2 Axial resolution

Fig. 1.3 Lateral resolution

axillary block, the ultrasound beam has to clearly distinguish between the axillary artery, axillary veins, the median, radial and ulnar nerves as well the muscle layer and fasciae.

Temporal Resolution The word temporal is derived from the Latin root 'tempus' which means time. Temporal resolution is the ability to precisely locate moving structures at given time instants. This has an important role in cardiological imaging. It depends on the processing speed and refresh rate of the ultrasound machine.

1.4 Interactions of Ultrasound with Tissue

The ultrasound wave is subjected to a number of interactions as it travels through a medium. These are (Fig. 1.4)

- Reflection
- Transmission
- Attenuation
- Scattering

Reflection

Reflection is the phenomenon in which a part of the energy is sent back to the medium from which the energy originates (Fig. 1.5).

Like all electromagnetic waves, sound waves also exhibit the phenomenon of reflection. The amount of reflection from a surface depends on the angle of incidence and the difference of impedances between two media.

There is an absence of echo/reflection if there is no difference in media impedances. However, in an interface between lung or bone and soft tissues, there is a significant difference between the media impedances which results in the creation of strong echoes.

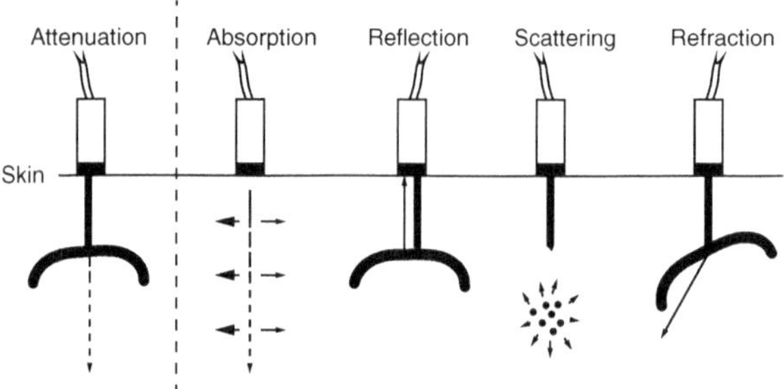

Fig. 1.4 Interaction of ultrasound with tissue

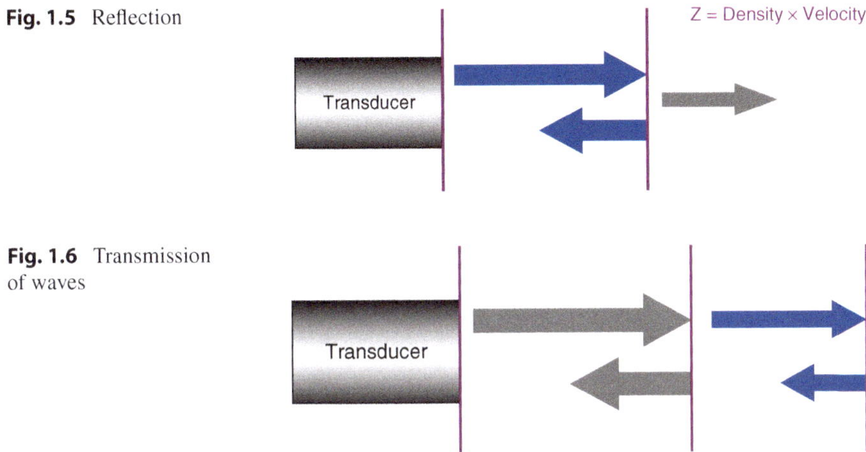

Fig. 1.5 Reflection

Fig. 1.6 Transmission of waves

Ultrasound is almost totally reflected at the interface between tissue/liquid and air, producing the brightest echo. E.g. the echo produced by pleura in a normal lung.

Refraction is the change of direction of sound while crossing the interface between two media. The radiological significance of this phenomenon is the creation of artefacts such as those seen under larger vessels on USG.

Transmission

Not all waves are reflected when passing through dissimilar media, some are transmitted (Fig. 1.6). The transmitted waves generally produce a weaker echo, therefore with increasing depth the amplitude and resolution of ultrasound weakens.

Attenuation

The amplitude of the sound waves decreases with increasing depth of penetration in the body. This is known as attenuation. It happens due to the loss of the sound energy. Lost energy is absorbed by the medium producing heat. The loss of energy, and thus attenuation is directly related to the frequency of the ultrasound beam.

Thus, the greater the frequency, the more the attenuation, and lesser is the penetration of the ultrasound wave.

Attenuation coefficient is a measure of attenuation caused by each tissue as a function of the ultrasound wave frequency. The practical aspect of this, for example, is that tissues such as bones have a high attenuation coefficient which greatly limits the transmission of ultrasound beam. Also, this means penetration shall decrease with increasing frequency.

Scattering This is the redirection of sound waves in different directions caused due to interaction with a rough surface or small reflector (Fig. 1.7).

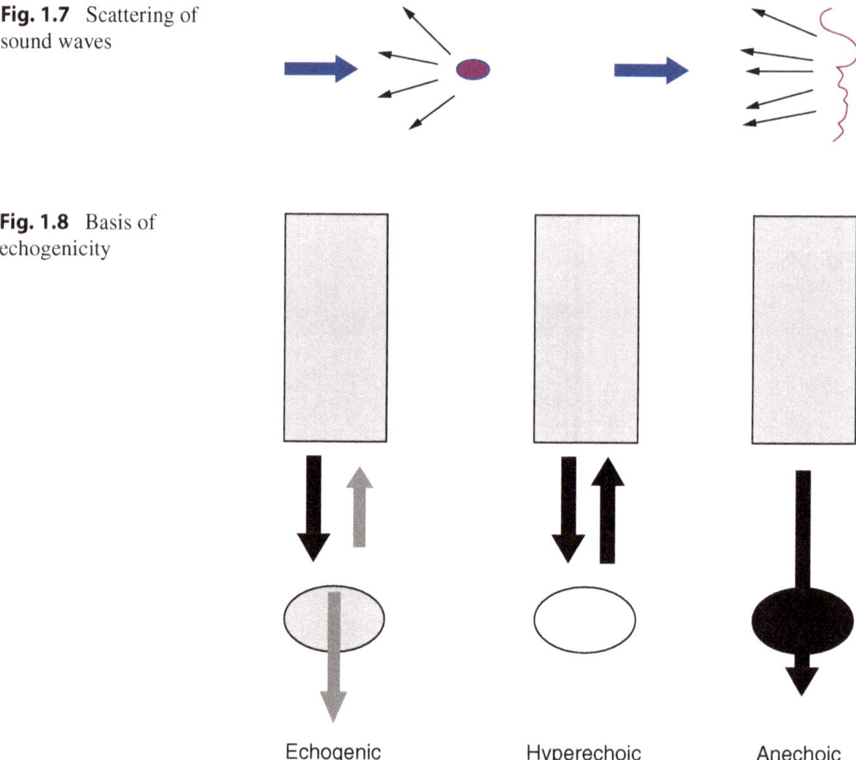

Fig. 1.7 Scattering of sound waves

Fig. 1.8 Basis of echogenicity

1.5 Echogenicity

The ultrasound waves reflected by tissues return to the transducer to produce an image. This phenomenon is similar to echoes that we hear in an empty hall. The property of tissues to generate echo is called echogenicity (Figs. 1.8 and 1.9).

The tissue which produces a similar echo to its surrounding tissue is called isoechoic, the tissue that causes lesser echo hypoechoic, e.g. muscles, the tissue that causes more echo is called hyperechoic, e.g. fascia, bones, pleura; the tissue that produces minimal or no echo is called anechoic, e.g. liquid filled cavity such as blood vessels, pleural effusion, etc.

Modes of Imaging

Although medical ultrasound began with A-mode, gradually more and more complex modes have been added. The mode most commonly used in regional anaesthesia practice is B-mode, which is also known as 2D ultrasound. Table 1.1 summarises different modes of ultrasound in medical imaging.

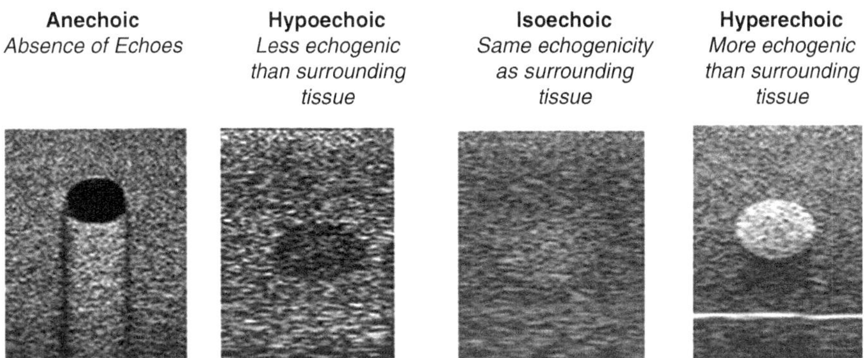

Fig. 1.9 Basis of echogenicity—anechoic, hypoechoic, isoechoic and hyperechoic tissues

Table 1.1 Modes of imaging

A-Mode	This is the most basic mode and works by displaying the reflected sound pulses on a time axis from a single line scan. This mode is not of much use in clinical anaesthesia.
B-Mode	This is a 2-D version of the A-mode and the most popularly used mode in anaesthesia. On passing through a slice of tissue, the reflected ultrasound beam is displayed which depicts the anatomical cross-section.
M-Mode	This mode can detect the movement of reflecting media along a single line scan. Often used along with the B-mode, this mode is popularly used in cardiological imaging to visualise heart valve movement.
Doppler Mode	This mode is based on the Doppler effect which is described by a change in the frequency of sound due to the relative motion between the source and receiver of sound. In this mode, the reflected sound waves, when ultrasonic waves are beamed along an artery or vein, have a Doppler change in frequency due to the motion of blood.
Colour Doppler	This provides a colour-coded image of Doppler shifts. The direction of blood flow depends on the direction of motion towards or away from the transducer. By convention, red and blue colours are selected for identification of direction and velocity of the blood.
Power Doppler	Nearly five times more sensitive than colour Doppler and is used to scan smaller vessels more accurately. This mode, however, does not provide any information on the speed and direction of flow.

1.6 Transducers

The ultrasound transducer, commonly called 'probe' is the part held by the operators hand that come in contact with the patient. It is a vital part of the machine as it contains the PE crystals that emit and receive ultrasound. Transducers come in various sizes and shapes. The shape of a probe governs the field of vision while the frequency of sound waves emitted governs the image resolution and depth of penetration (Fig. 1.10).

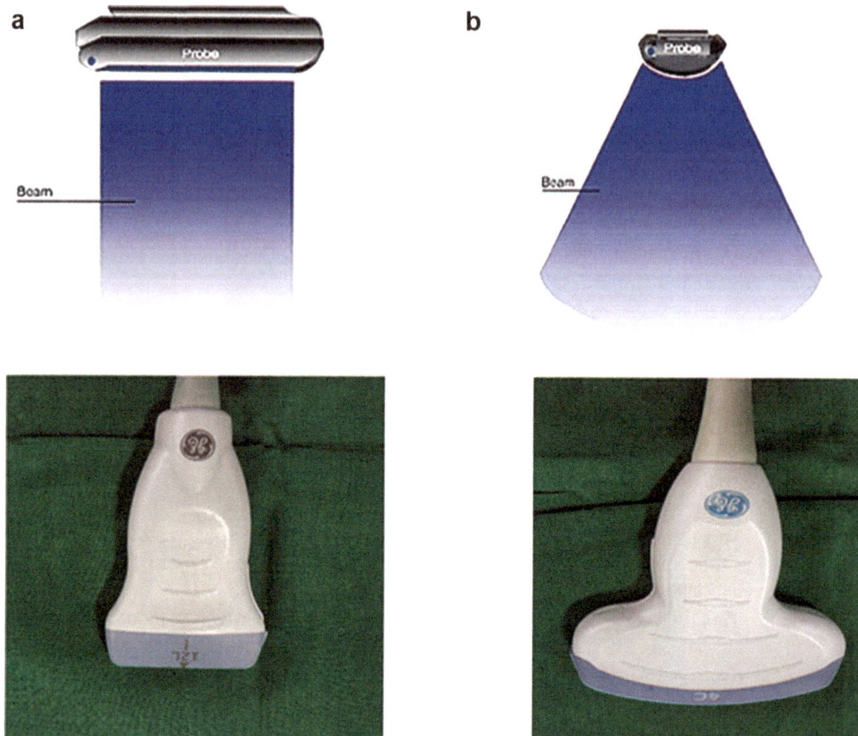

Fig. 1.10 (**a**) Linear and (**b**) Curvilinear transducers and their ultrasound beam pattern

The linear probe emits a linear array of ultrasound and produces a rectangular image. It is usually of high frequency and low penetration. The higher frequency gives the linear probe better image resolution and is favoured for superficial interventions where high accuracy is required.

The curvilinear probe emits a curved array of the ultrasound beam and produces a curved image. It has a lower frequency but a wider area of imaging and greater depth. Due to low frequency, the image resolution is grainy and inferior compared to a linear probe. However, for deeper blocks, imaging and interventions it is the transducer of choice.

1.7 Time Gain Compensation

This is an operator-controlled amplification technique to make up for the sound attenuation as ultrasound waves travel through tissue. It must be manually adjusted for each tissue type to be scanned and manipulated for best image optimisation.

The TGC control layout differs from one machine to another. The presence of slider knobs is a popular design; each knob in the slider set controls the gain for a specific depth, which gives a well-balanced image (Fig. 1.11). Accordingly, the sliders are called near field TGC and far-field TGC.

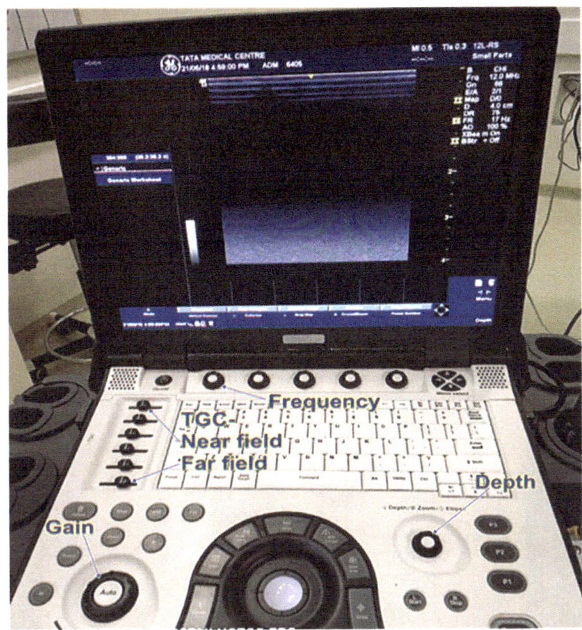

Fig. 1.11 The TGC layout in a standard USG machine

1.8 Practical Aspects

The ultimate objective of learning the basics of ultrasound imaging is to be able to obtain an optimal image. For image optimization, the following points should be kept in mind [7–9]:

- Frequency of the transducer
- Depth adjustment
- Gain
- Focus
- Compound imaging use (Fig. 1.12)

Frequency Higher frequency is usually selected for superficial interventions that require greater resolution. With decreasing frequency, tissues at greater depth can be imaged, at the cost of resolution (Fig. 1.13).

Depth Depth of the image has to be adjusted to the depth of the object to be blocked or the depth of the intervention endpoint. The depth selected should be at least a few centimetres more than the depth of the target. That way, if the needle overshoots the target it can be seen. Also, the nearby anatomical structures would remain visible.

Decreasing the depth increases magnification and vice versa. For superficial blocks, by decreasing depth setting, greater details can be appreciated.

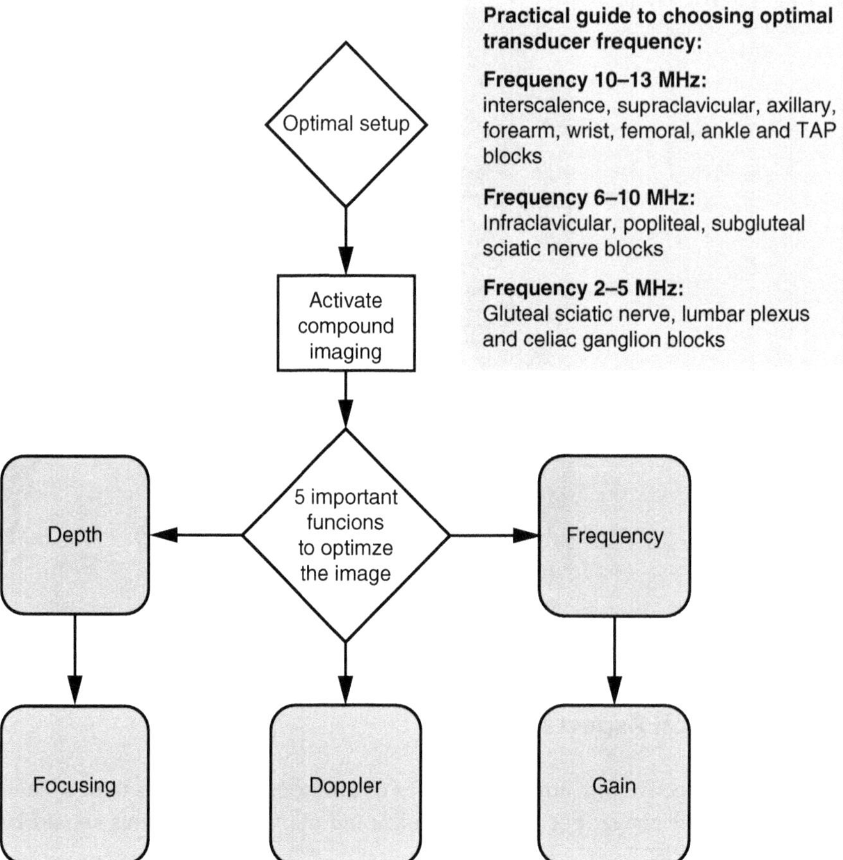

Fig. 1.12 Algorithm for optimum imaging with ultrasound

Gain The gain function is used to increase overall screen brightness. An optimum gain should be used to obtain the best possible contrast between the muscles and the connective tissue (fascia) for a nerve block because usually the nerves produce echo that is similar to the connective tissue. While TGC controls are used to modify the gain at different depths, overall gain can be adjusted using the gain button (Fig. 1.14).

Focus Focus of the ultrasound image is the narrowest point of the ultrasound beam. It is the point where the image resolution is best. Modern ultrasound machines have electronic focus adjustment capacity. It is best to place the focus just at the level of or slightly below the object to be viewed for optimum image quality.

The ultrasound machine *console* (Fig. 1.15) contains the buttons and sliders for modifying all the above factors such as frequency, depth, focus, etc. One must be well versed with the console to obtain the best image and to be able to store and retrieve images.

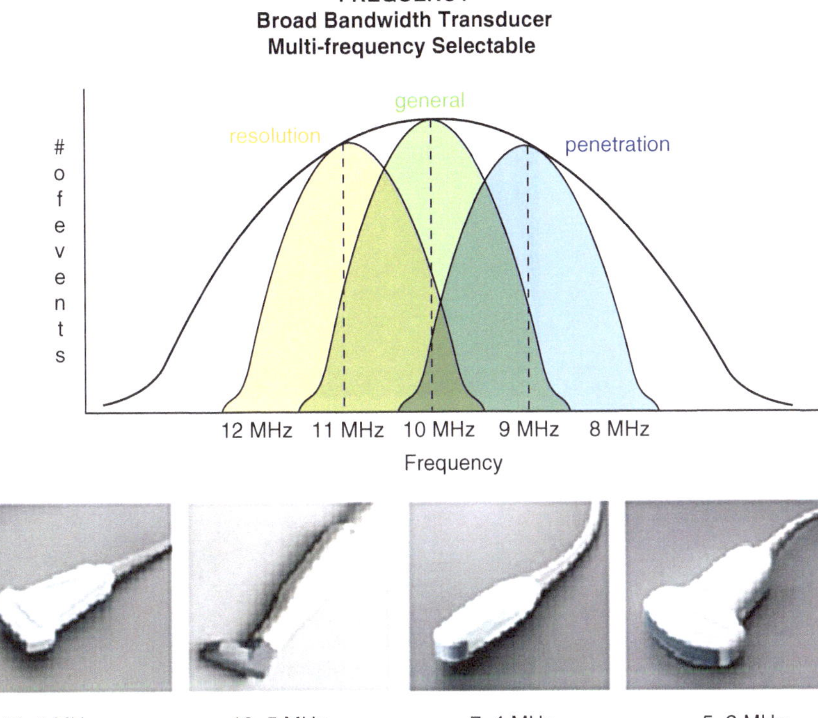

Fig. 1.13 Frequency and transducers

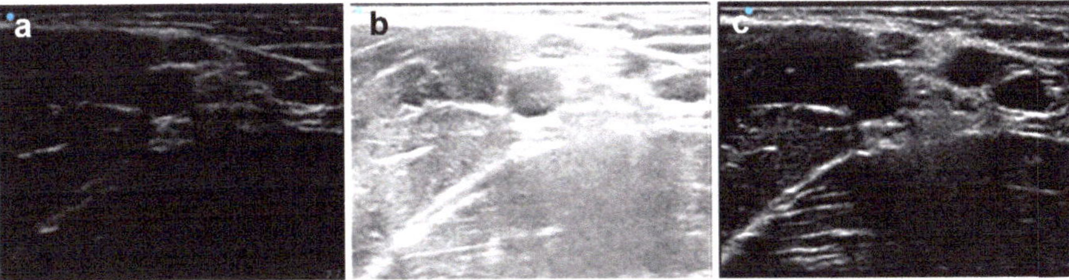

Fig. 1.14 Gain adjustment: ultrasound scan of the axillary area with the gain adjustment: (**a**) low gain, (**b**) high gain, (**c**) optimal gain

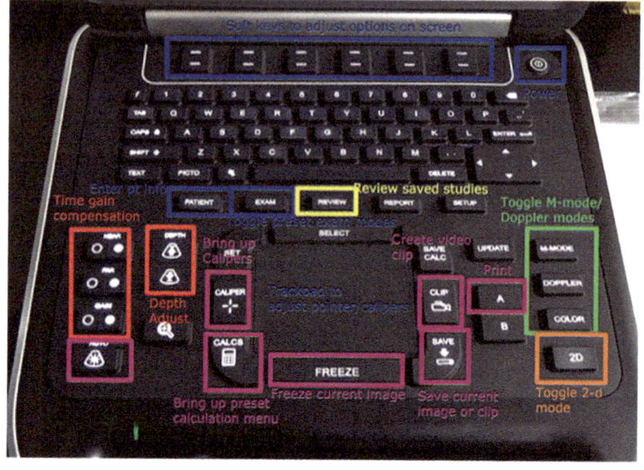

Fig. 1.15 US console showing frequently used functions

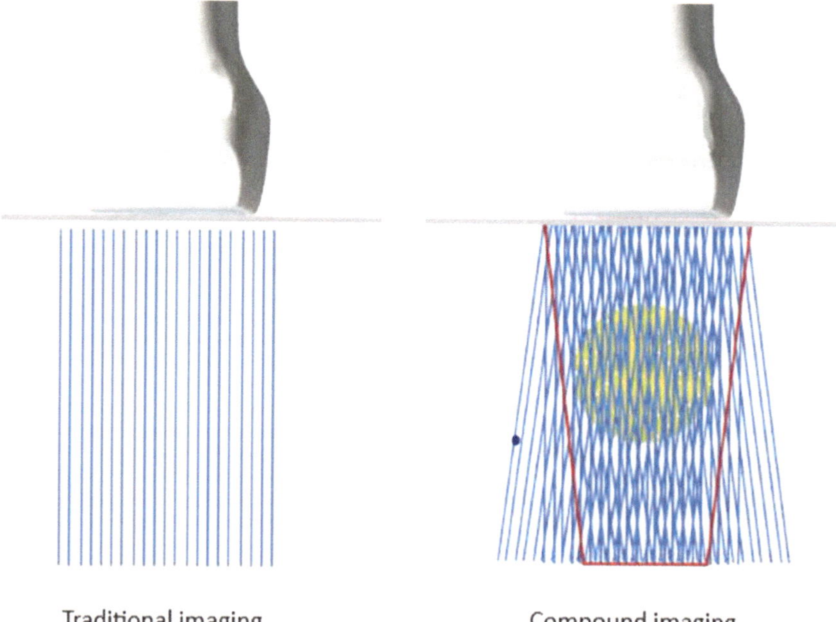

Fig. 1.16 Compound image combines multiple coplanar images with images obtained from multiple frequency spectra to form a single image

1.9 Compound Imaging

It is the technology that combines multiple coplanar images (spatial compounding) with images obtained from multiple frequency spectra (frequency compounding) to form a single image. This decreases artefacts and speckles and improves resolution [10] (Fig. 1.16).

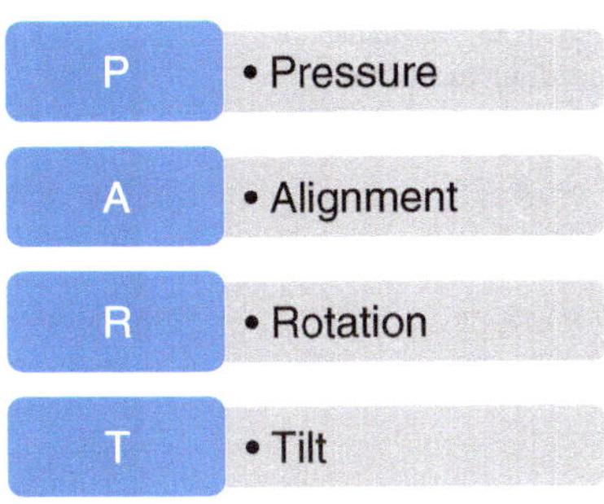

Fig. 1.17 PART manoeuvre to obtain optimal image

1.10 Manoeuvring the US Probe: PART

Even after optimising the image setting, optimal image may not be obtained. For that, the ultrasound probe needs to be held and manoeuvred (Fig. 1.17).

Pressure By putting mild pressure with the probe, subcutaneous fat can be displaced and a better image can be obtained.

Alignment Proper alignment of the probe in the recommended plane is required to obtain clinically useful image. E.g. the US probe is held transversely for a TAP block, but sagitally for an SAP block.

Rotation The probe may need to be slightly rotated to align it perfectly with the underlying tissue and the block needle. E.g. for supraclavicular brachial plexus block, the probe needs to be slightly externally rotated.

Tilt Slight cephalad, caudal, lateral, medial or oblique tilt may be necessary for the optimal image. Because of the direction of the nerve fibres, some nerves seem different at different angles and a little tilt is required to obtain the perpendicular cross-section and hence the best image. This property of tissues is called *anisotropy*. E.g. caudal tilt is required for imaging the supraclavicular brachial plexus.

1.11 Needling Techniques

The Ultrasound beam travels in a straight line, like a thin sheet, perpendicular to the probe. How the intervening needle is visualised depends on how much of its length is in alignment with the ultrasound beam [11, 12].

In Plane

The needle is placed parallel to the transducer. The needle shaft and tip are both visible (Figs. 1.18 and 1.19).

Example: axillary block.

This approach is safe and easy to learn but is difficult to practice in deeper blocks. The quality of needle visualisation depends on the angle of entry of the needle.

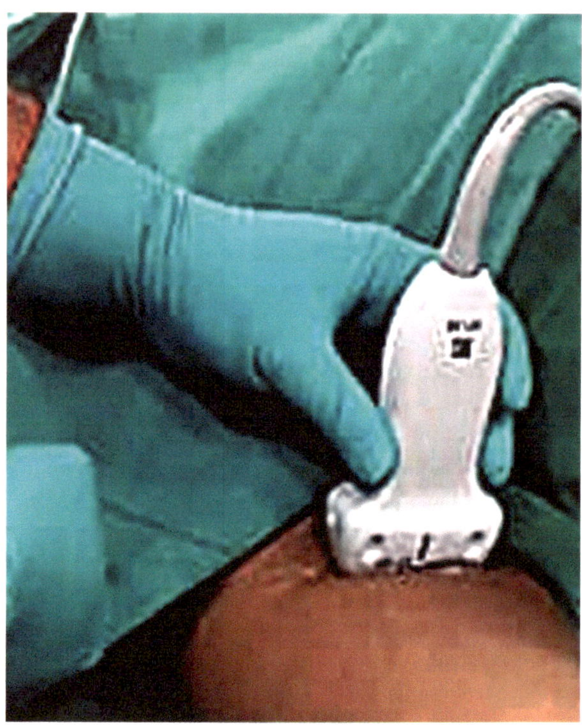

Fig. 1.18 In plane needling technique

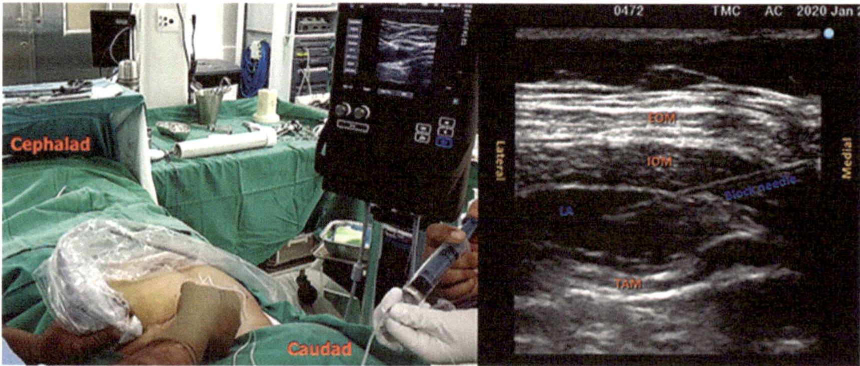

Fig. 1.19 In plane needling technique. Note that the entire length of the needle and its tip is imaged in real time

Flatter the angle (acute angle), the better is the image. To reach deeper objects, a more perpendicular angle is required, which makes needle visualisation in this technique difficult.

Out of Plane

The needle is placed perpendicular to the transducer probe. The tip of the needle may be difficult to locate accurately in this approach and the use of echogenic tip

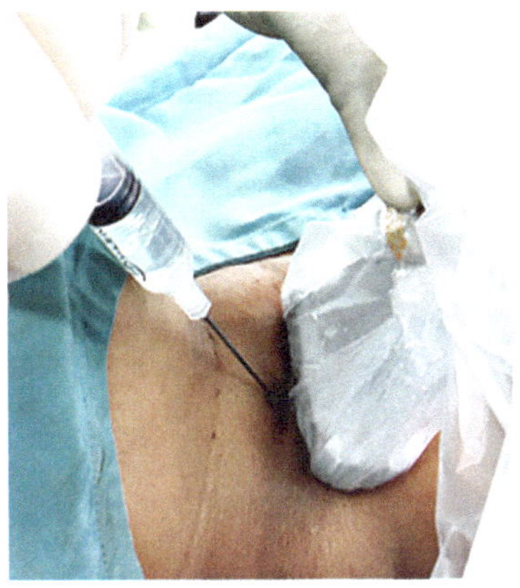

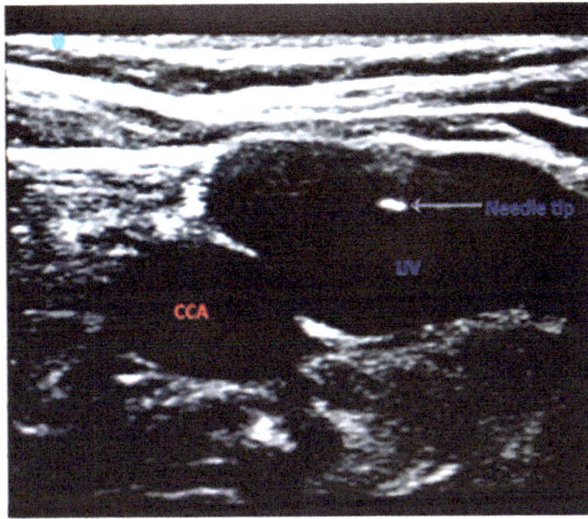

Fig. 1.20 Out of plane cannulation of internal jugular vein (IJV): Left panel shows the probe holding and needle entering out of the plane at a right angle to the probe. The ultrasound image on the right shows the sonoanatomy and the tip of the needle being seen as a bright hyperechoic spot. *CCA* common carotid artery lies medial to the IJV

needles is advised. *It is important to observe tissue displacement by the advancing needle tip as often the needle tip may not be seen.*

For superficial procedures such as internal jugular vein cannulation, it is a good strategy to estimate the depth of the target and calculate the entry point of the needle, angle of inclination and angle of the ultrasound probe accordingly. For deeper structures, hydrodissection with 1–2 ml saline can be used to conform the location of the needle tip.

Actual needle to nerve contact can be verified by nerve stimulation and pattern of local anaesthetic spread.

Example: Femoral nerve block, vascular cannulations (Fig. 1.20).

1.12 Bioeffect and Safety

Ultrasound application produces biologic effect by thermal and non-thermal mechanisms. Heat is generated through the absorption of ultrasound by tissues and is directly proportional to ultrasound intensity, frequency and duration.

Two standard indices are displayed by an ultrasound machine (Fig. 1.21)

Thermal Index (TI) It is the transducer acoustic power divided by the estimated power needed to increase tissue temperature by 1 degree.

Mechanical Index (MI) It is the peak rarefactional pressure divided by the square root of the centre frequency of the pulse bandwidth. The relative likelihood of thermal and mechanical hazard is indicated by TI and MI, respectively. TI or MI >1.0 is dangerous.

Different tissue and examination setting are saved and categorised in modern ultrasound machines to aid in imaging as well as reducing these bioeffects. For

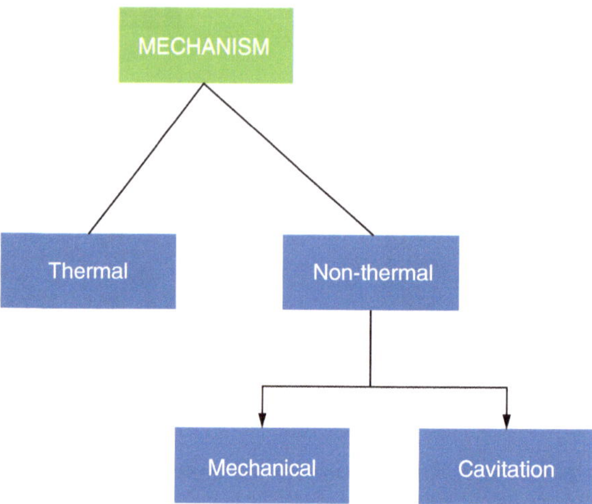

Fig. 1.21 Bioeffect and safety

example, the ophthalmic mode is a low power setting that allows examination of the eyes without causing any tissue injury to the sensitive ophthalmic tissues such as the retina.

Artefacts Artefacts are false images produced due to highly reflective tissue interfaces. There are various types of artefacts, such as comet tail artefact, mirror image artefacts, etc.

Some of the artefacts are misleading, whereas some are useful. Lung ultrasound artefacts such as A lines and B lines are pathognomonic and useful for the detection of clinical conditions.

These artefacts are described in detail in textbooks of point of care ultrasound.

1.13 Blockmate Pearls

Knowledge of ultrasound physics is needed for image optimization. The key understandings are

- Appropriate transducer selection
- Gain Settings
- Depth Settings
- Tissue Echo Characteristics
- Ultrasound Artefacts

For optimal imaging, it is important to adjust the *pressure, alignment, rotation and tilt* (PART) of the probe.

The best needle image is obtained when the needle forms an acute angle with the ultrasound probe as more US waves reflect off the needle. The more steep the angle, the lesser is the needle visibility. The best image is produced by a needle that is parallel to the ultrasound probe, i.e. perpendicular to the ultrasound beam.

For deeper tissues, it is useful to enter the needle 2–3 cm away from the edge of the ultrasound probe so that a reasonably acute angle can be formed.

References

1. Marhofer P, Chan VW. Ultrasound-guided regional anesthesia: current concepts and future trends. Anesth Analg. 2007;104:1265–9.
2. Neal JM, Brull R, Chan VW, Grant SA, Horn JL, Liu SS, et al. The ASRA evidence-based medicine assessment of ultrasound-guided regional anesthesia and pain medicine. Executive summary. Reg Anesth Pain Med. 2010;35:S1–9.
3. Cory PC. Concerns regarding ultrasound-guided regional anesthesia. Anesthesiology. 2009;111:1167–8.
4. Brull R, Macfarlane AJ, Tse CC. Practical knobology for ultrasound-guided regional anesthesia. Reg Anesth Pain Med. 2010;35:S68–73.
5. Merritt CR. Physics of ultrasound. In: Rumack CM, Wilson SR, Charboneau JA, editors. Diagnostic ultrasound. 3rd ed. St. Louis: Elsevier Mosby; 2005.
6. Sites BD, Brull R, Chan VW, Spence BC, Gallagher J, Beach ML, et al. Artifacts and pitfall errors associated with ultrasound-guided regional anesthesia. Part II: A pictorial approach to understanding and avoidance. Reg Anesth Pain Med. 2007;32:419–33.
7. Bigeleisen PE, editor. Ultrasound-guided regional anesthesia and pain medicine. London: Lippincott Williams and Wilkins; 2010.
8. Pollard BA, Chan VW. Introductory curriculum for ultrasound-guided regional anesthesia. Toronto: University of Toronto Press; 2009.
9. Tsui BC. Atlas of ultrasound and nerve stimulation-guided regional anesthesia. New York: Springer Science+Business Media; 2007.
10. Brian DS, Macfarlane AJ, Sites VR, Chan VW, Brull R, et al. Clinical sonopathology for the regional anesthesiologist. Reg Anesth Pain Med. 2010;35:272–89.
11. Maecken T, Zenz M, Grau T. Ultrasound characteristics of needles for regional anesthesia. Reg Anesth Pain Med. 2007;32:440–7.
12. Pollard BA. New model for learning ultrasound-guided needle to target localization. Reg Anesth Pain Med. 2008;33:360–2.

Regional Anaesthesia for the Upper Limb

2

Arunangshu Chakraborty and Anshuman Sarkar

2.1 Introduction

Brachial plexus block at the supraclavicular level and at the axillary level is one of the oldest practised regional anaesthesia techniques. A well-established brachial plexus block produces surgical anaesthesia with muscle relaxation and reliable postoperative analgesia. With the use of ultrasound, the upper limb blocks have become more predictable, reliable and safe. In this chapter, we will describe each of the block techniques in a sequential manner and enumerate their clinical applications. It is important to remember the anatomical landmarks and structures underneath while performing the blocks.

Anatomy The upper limb is innervated mostly from the branches of the brachial plexus (BrP) apart from a small area in the medial aspect of the upper arm which is supplied by the intercostobrachial nerve that has a root from the second thoracic intercostal nerve and upper part of the shoulder that is supplied by the supraclavicular nerve (C3-4). While deciding for a block, it is important to remember that the skin innervation may be different from the muscle or bone. Accordingly dermatome, myotome and osteotome distributions should be learned for a successful regional anaesthesia practice (Figs. 2.1, 2.2, and 2.3).

The brachial plexus is formed by the anterior rami of the spinal nerves C5 (fifth cervical) to T1 (first thoracic) (Fig. 2.2). Occasionally C4 (pre-fixed BrP) or T2 (post-fixed BrP) may contribute to the formation of the plexus. C5 and C6 roots join to form the upper trunk, C7 is continued as the middle trunk and C8 and T1 combine

A. Chakraborty (✉)
Department of Anaesthesia, CC and Pain, Tata Medical Center, Kolkata, India

A. Sarkar
Tata Medical Center, Kolkata, India
e-mail: anshuman.sarkar@tmckolkata.com

A. Chakraborty (ed.), *Blockmate*, https://doi.org/10.1007/978-981-15-9202-7_2

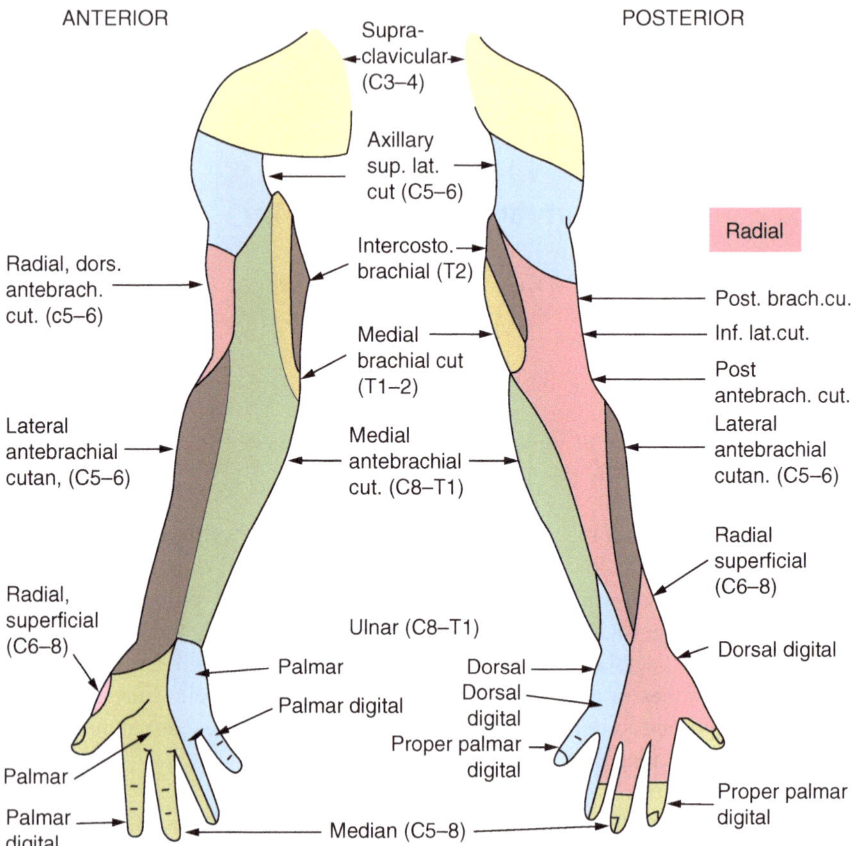

Fig. 2.1 Cutaneous innervation of the upper limb (dermatome). This is a digitally retouched render of a Wikimedia commons file. URL: https://en.wikipedia.org/wiki/File:Gray812and814.svg. Digitally modified by Dr. Arunangshu Chakraborty

to form the lower trunk. Each trunk is then divided into anterior and posterior divisions. Anterior divisions of the upper and middle trunks combine to form the lateral cord, anterior division of the lower trunk continues as the medial cord and posterior division of all the three trunks combine to form the posterior cord. Individual nerves originate from the roots, trunks, divisions and cords (Table 2.1).

In the axilla bulk of the lateral and medial cords unite to form the median nerve, which is the most prominent nerve of the upper limb, the posterior cord is continued as the radial nerve and the medial cord as the ulnar nerve.

While performing blocks, it is important to remember and correlate with this anatomy that the interscalene block, which is the highest (most proximal) block of the brachial plexus blocks the trunks, generally the upper and middle. The nerves

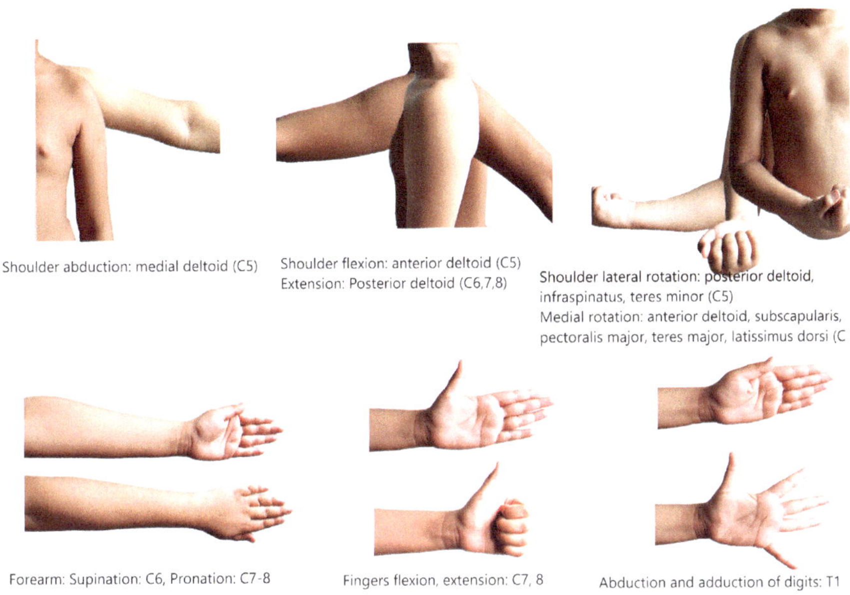

Fig. 2.2 Muscular innervation of the upper limb (Myotome)

that appear from the C5 root such as the dorsal scapular and the area innervated by the lower trunk are likely to be spared with an interscalene block. Similarly, the supraclavicular perivascular block that approaches the plexus at the divisions level would spare the dorsal scapular, nerve to subclavius and suprascapular nerves. The axillary block would miss all the nerves rising from the roots, trunks and divisions (Fig. 2.4).

One important yet common complication of the brachial plexus block is the hemidiaphragmatic palsy caused by the block of the phrenic nerve. As the phrenic nerve (C3-5) lies anterior to the anterior scalene muscle (ASM) and travels from lateral to the medial border of ASM to eventually enter the thorax between the subclavian artery and vein, even a small volume of local anaesthetic injected at the C5/C6 level for interscalene block would affect it. Even with the supraclavicular perivascular approach, the incidence is about 67%. The infraclavicular approach reduces the incidence of phrenic palsy, but the block is technically challenging and fraught with the risk of accidental pneumothorax. Axillary block may be safest from the phrenic palsy perspective, but it often spares the radial nerve and branches of the posterior cord along with musculocutaneous nerve, therefore not being popular for surgery at or above the elbow. One recently described technique, the costoclavicular block provides excellent analgesia while causing less phrenic blockade compared to

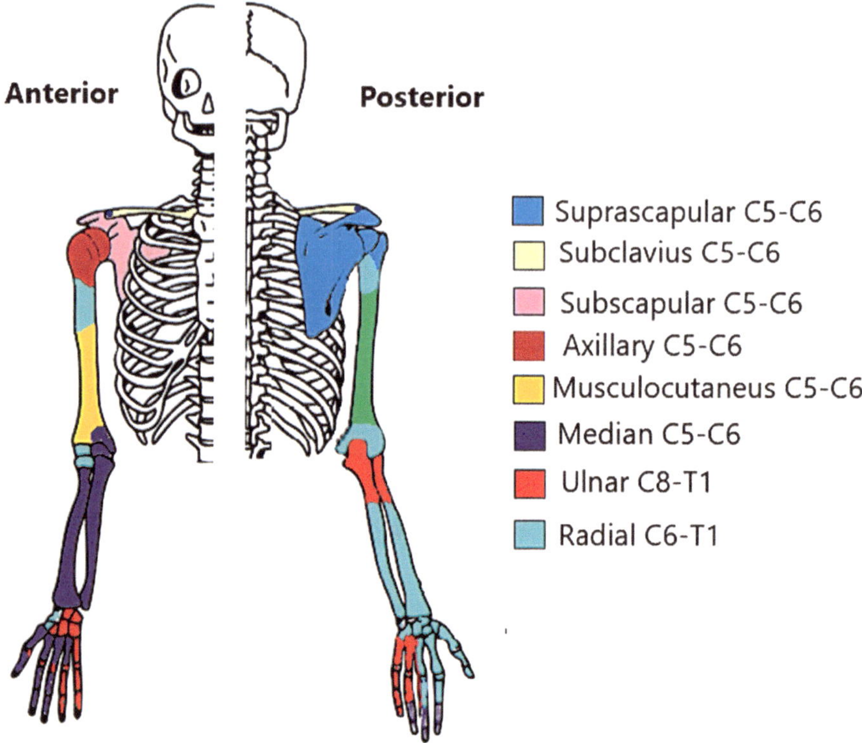

Fig. 2.3 Osteotomes of the upper limb

Table 2.1 Branches of brachial plexus

Specific region of the brachial plexus	Branches arising from the brachial plexus
Roots	Nerve to longus cervicis (C5–8) Nerve to the scalene muscles (C5–8) Nerve to rhomboids (C5) Nerve to serratus anterior (C5–7) contribution to the phrenic nerve (C5)
Trunks	Nerve to subclavius (C5, 6) Suprascapular nerve (C5, 6)
Lateral cord	Lateral pectoral nerve (C5–7) Musculocutaneous nerve (C5–7) Lateral head of median nerve (C6, 7)
Medial cord	Medial pectoral nerve (C8, T1) Medial cutaneous nerve of arm (C8, T1) Medial cutaneous nerve of forearm (C8, T1) Medial head of median nerve (C8, T1) Ulnar nerve (C7–8, T1)
Posterior cord	Upper subscapular nerve (C5, 6) Nerve to latissimus dorsi (thoracodorsal nerve) (C6–8) Lower subscapular nerve (C5, 6) Axillary nerve (C5, 6) Radial nerve (C5–8, T1)

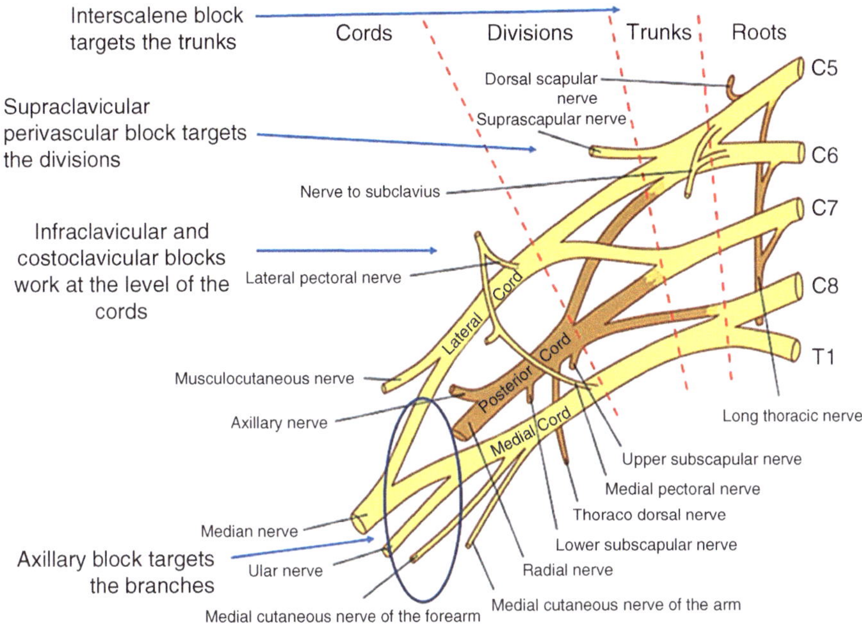

Fig. 2.4 Formation of brachial plexus and levels of blocks. This is a digitally retouched render of a Wikimedia commons file. URL: https://en.wikipedia.org/wiki/File:Brachial_plexus_2.svg. Digitally modified by Dr. Arunangshu Chakraborty. Original image description: Anterior view of right brachial plexus. Illustration. Modified by Mattopaedia on 02-Jan-2006 from the 1918 Edition of Gray's Anatomy. Original unmodified image sourced from http://www.bartleby.com/107. Migrated to vector (.svg) image on 11-November-2009 by Captain-n00dle. Simplified image on 30-November-2009 by MissMJ

the supraclavicular perivascular approach. However, unlike the supraclavicular or infraclavicular technique, costoclavicular block cannot be performed without ultrasound guidance (Fig. 2.5).

Blockmate Pearls

- Although there are seven cervical vertebrae (C1-C7), there are eight cervical nerves C1–C8. All cervical nerves except C8 emerge above their corresponding vertebrae, while the C8 nerve emerges below the C7 vertebra. Elsewhere in the spine, the nerve emerges below the vertebra with the same name.
- The supraclavicular branches of brachial plexus are the branches from the roots and trunks of the plexus that arise in the neck, but the major distribution of the plexus is derived from its infraclavicular branches.

Equipments for Block:

- Ultrasound machine with high-frequency linear transducer
- Local anaesthetic (LA)
- 100 mm, 22G, short bevel, echogenic needle with nerve stimulation

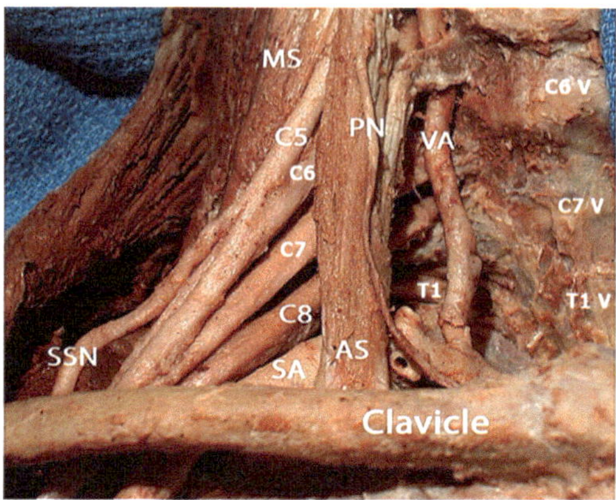

Fig. 2.5 Cadaveric dissection of the brachial plexus: Note the nerve roots C5–C8, vertebral artery (VA) exposed at the levels of C7 and T1 vertebrae, the anterior (AS) and middle (MS) scalene muscles forming the scalene groove that is the outlet and the anatomical landmark for the brachial plexus. The suprascapular nerve (SSN) is seen arising from the upper trunk. The subclavian artery (SA) lies deep to the clavicle and the anterior scalene muscle. The perivascular approach for the brachial plexus would be lateral to the artery as seen. The phrenic nerve (PN) lies anterior to the anterior scalene muscle and as such would be most affected by the interscalene block and least by the axillary

- Peripheral nerve stimulator
- Syringes
- Camera cover
- Coupling gel
- Sterile drape and skin disinfectant solution
- Sterile 5% dextrose solution

2.2 Block Techniques

2.2.1 The Interscalene Block

Patient Position The patient lies with his head turned to the other side and arms adducted (Fig. 2.6). A beach chair position can be used as well. Elevation of the head end improves patient comfort and venous drainage of neck veins and thereby bleeding.

Scanning Technique Ultrasound transducer is placed in a transverse orientation above the transverse process of the sixth cervical vertebra (C6), which usually corresponds with the cricoid cartilage. While scanning from medial to lateral, structures such as the cricoid cartilage, the thyroid gland, the common carotid artery, the internal jugular vein, the anterior scalene muscle, the cervical nerve roots and the middle scalene muscle are seen (Fig. 2.7). A little caudal tilt improves the cross-

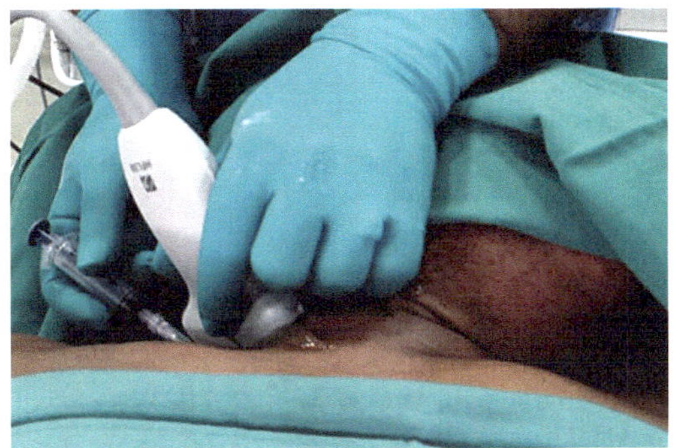

Fig. 2.6 Patient and probe position for an interscalene block

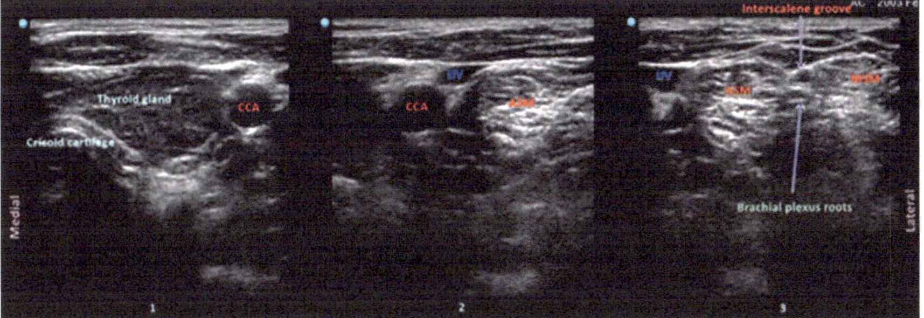

Fig. 2.7 Ultrasound scanning for interscalene block: The scan starts medially from the easy landmark of the common carotid artery (CCA) and proceeds laterally identifying landmarks such as the internal jugular vein (IJV), anterior scalene muscle (ASM) and middle scalene muscle (MSM). In between the two scalene muscles, the interscalene groove and the roots of brachial plexus can be identified

sectional image of the nerve roots. C5, C6 and C7 roots can be easily seen coming out of the groove between the anterior and posterior tubercles of the transverse processes of respective vertebrae. The anterior tubercle of the C6 is bigger than the posterior tubercle and is a distinctive feature. Immediately above the anterior tubercle of C5 is usually smaller than the posterior tubercle and below at the C7 level, the anterior tubercle is absent, where the vertebral artery can be seen instead as it enters the transverse foramen of C6. Typically, the plexus is seen like a 'traffic light' with the C5, C6 and C7 roots in the cross-section being aligned in the same plane (Fig. 2.8).

Injection Endpoint Target of this block is to inject local anaesthetic around the brachial plexus components located between the anterior and middle scalene muscles. Spread of the LA around the nerve roots is visualised under ultrasound in real time. After identifying the roots injection can be given superficial to C5, between C5 and C6 or deep to C6. Injection between C6 and 7 is better avoided for the fear of intraneural injection.

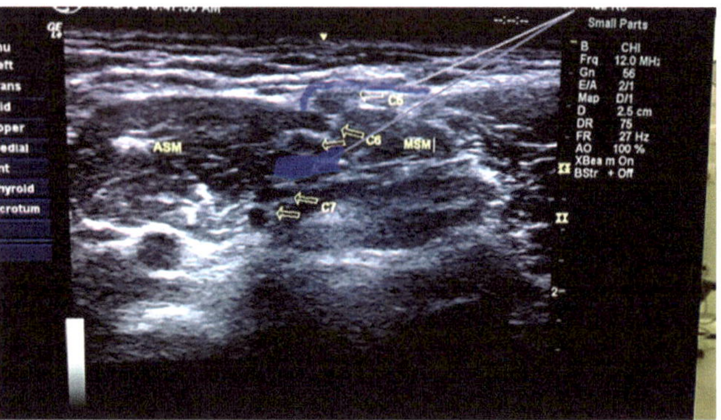

Fig. 2.8 Sonoanatomy of interscalene area: Note the anterior scalene muscle (ASM), middle scalene muscle (MSM) and the brachial plexus roots lying in the interscalene groove in the typical 'traffic lights' fashion. The arrow represents the needle trajectory for the block

Block Technique After cleansing with antiseptic and draping, the area is scanned with ultrasound to identify the anatomical structures. One to two ml of local anaesthetic is injected at the point of entry. The needle is typically inserted from lateral to medial direction and is visualised 'in-plane'. A 'pop' is felt after piercing the prevertebral fascia. 1–2 ml LA is injected here to facilitate further needle advancement. For an out-of-plane approach the needle enters vertically along the mid point of the ultrasound transducer in a cephalo-caudad direction. Care should be taken that the needle does not go too close to the nerve roots as nerve injury from pressure effects are possible if the injection is nearer to the transverse foramen. Ten to fifteen ml of LA is usually sufficient for an adequate block. One injection in the interscalene groove at the level of C6 is usually adequate. A distal injection at C8-T1 level can be attempted for surgery around or below the elbow. Injection should be preferably superficial. Too deep injection tends to be interfascicular or intraneural. Pressure of injection should be carefully monitored. High pressure of injection indicates an intraneural position of the tip of the needle. As the area is highly vascular, frequent aspiration and injection in aliquots of 2–3 ml help to prevent intravascular injection.

Tips and Tricks Forward tracing starting at the transverse process and nerve roots to the plexus in the interscalene groove or backtracing from a supraclavicular position where the plexus is seen like a 'bunch of grapes' may be helpful in case it is difficult to locate the interscalene area. The common site of injection is at the level of C5-C6 nerve trunks. Adequate tracing of the nerve trunk distally can help identify the division of the trunks that can be commonly misinterpreted as separate nerve trunks.

Blockmate Pearls

- Interscalene block can sometimes cause Horner's syndrome, which is characterised by miosis (constriction of the pupil), ptosis (drooping of the eyelid) and anhydros (reduced sweating). It is usually transient and no treatment is needed as such.

- Ipsilateral hemidiaphragmatic palsy due to phrenic nerve blockade is commonly seen after an interscalene block. Patients with respiratory comorbidity might need oxygen supplementation. Interscalene block should not be administered bilaterally and better avoided in patients with moderate to severe COPD.
- A selective upper trunk block can be performed targeting only the fifth and sixth cervical nerve roots. It is useful for shoulder surgery where the block of the ulnar component is not required.

2.2.2 The Supraclavicular Perivascular Approach

Patient Position Similar to the interscalene block, the patient lies supine, head turned towards the opposite side, arms adducted. Placing a sandbag or sponge wedge below the shoulder or asking the patient to reach for the ipsilateral knee helps making the landmarks prominent and ultrasound imaging of the plexus.

Scanning Technique The scanning should start in the neck at the C6-7 level starting with the common carotid artery. After the common carotid artery is identified, the ultrasound probe is moved laterally to image the internal jugular vein, the sternomastoid muscle and the anterior scalene muscle followed by the elements of the brachial plexus in the interscalene groove. Once the interscalene groove is reached/ identified, the ultrasound probe is tilted caudally so that the ultrasound beam 'looks into the thorax'. In this location, the brachial plexus is seen like a 'bunch of grapes', lateral to the subclavian artery, medial to the middle scalene muscle. Below the brachial plexus the first rib and the pleura should be visible (Fig. 2.9).

Block Technique After cleansing with antiseptic and draping, the area is scanned with ultrasound identifying the anatomical structures and no fly zones such as the pleura and subclavian artery are located. One to two ml local anaesthetic is injected at the point of entry. The needle should be inserted from lateral to the medial direc-

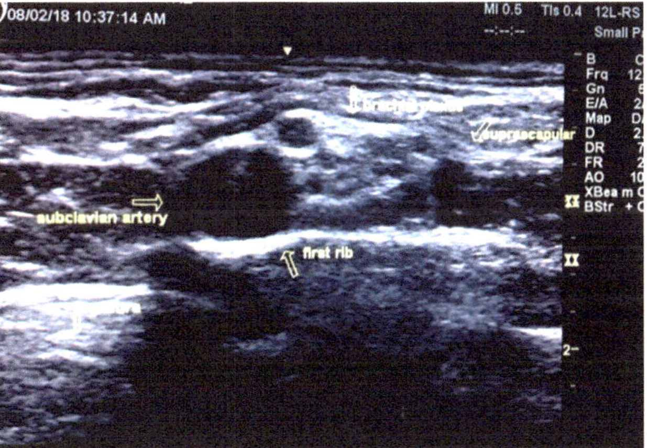

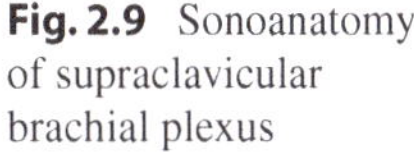
Fig. 2.9 Sonoanatomy of supraclavicular brachial plexus

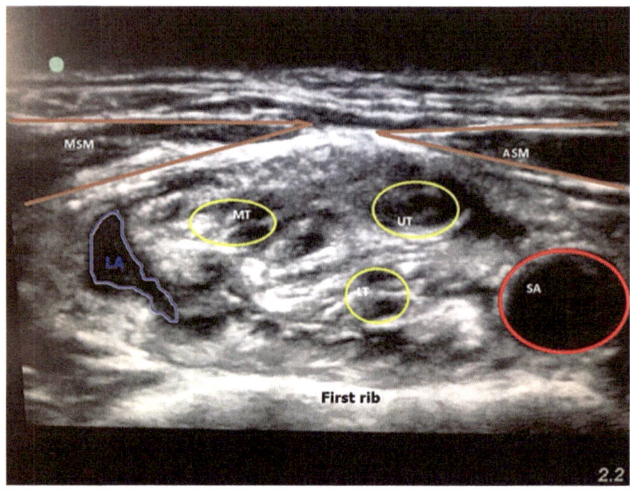

Fig. 2.10 Supraclavicular perivascular brachial plexus block: Note the subclavian artery (SA) and anterior scalene muscle (ASM) medial and the middle scalene lateral to the brachial plexus, identified as the upper (UT), middle (MT) and lower (LT) trunks. Note the local anaesthetic (LA) spread around the plexus

tion and advanced in plane to the ultrasound beam. For an out-of-plane approach, the needle enters vertically along the mid point of the ultrasound transducer in a cephalo-caudal orientation. Due to the nearness to the dome of the pleura, an out-of-plane approach has a higher risk of pneumothorax and is not recommended for beginners. Ideally an in plane 'corner pocket' injection at the 6 O' clock position of the plexus should be given first, followed by injection at 12 o' clock. After 10–15 ml injection LA is seen spread all around the brachial plexus in a typical 'donut' sign (Fig. 2.10).

It is important to keep the first rib and the pleura in the ultrasound image while inserting the needle to prevent pneumothorax.

High pressure of injection indicates an intraneural position of the tip of the needle. As the area is highly vascular, frequent aspiration and injection in aliquots of 2–3 ml help to prevent intravascular injection.

Indications
Surgery of the arm, elbow, forearm and hand

2.2.3 The Infraclavicular Approach

Position Patient lies supine with the ipsilateral arm abducted and flexed at elbow at 90 degrees. Care should be taken not to hyperabduct the arm. The arm should be rested over a padded arm board. The operator should stand at the head end of the patient with the ultrasound machine kept distal to the arm board directly facing the anaesthesiologist. Abduction pulls the clavicle upwards and brings the cords closer to the skin (Fig. 2.11).

Anatomical Landmark Coracoid process

Sonoanatomy The important sonoanatomy landmarks are

- Second part of axillary artery
- Axillary vein medial to artery
- Pectoralis major
- Pectoralis minor

Technique After positioning the patient and application of sterile dressing and draping ASA standard monitors are attached and intravenous access is obtained. Ultrasound transducer is placed parasagittally just medial to the coracoid process below the clavicle. During the scout scan it is important to identify pectoralis major and minor muscles, axillary artery (confirm with colour doppler showing pulsatile flow), axillary vein (confirm compressibility with transducer and with colour doppler showing continuous flow) and individual cords. Considering the axillary artery as the dial of a clock; the lateral cord usually lies between 10 o' clock to 8 o' clock position, the posterior cord between 7 o' clock to 4 o'clock position and the medial cord between artery and vein at 2 o'clock position. The depth of the field may need to be increased to identify the pleura. Scanning medially helps. The needle should approach from the cephalad side, in plane, the full length of the needle should be visible all the time.

- Initially target to bring the needle on the posterior aspect of the axillary artery to block the posterior cord—do not get confused between the cord and posterior acoustic enhancement. After careful aspiration, inject 1–2 ml of 5% dextrose for hydro dissection and confirm proper placement with nerve stimulation. Thereafter deposit small aliquots of LA and observe for U shaped distribution of LA around

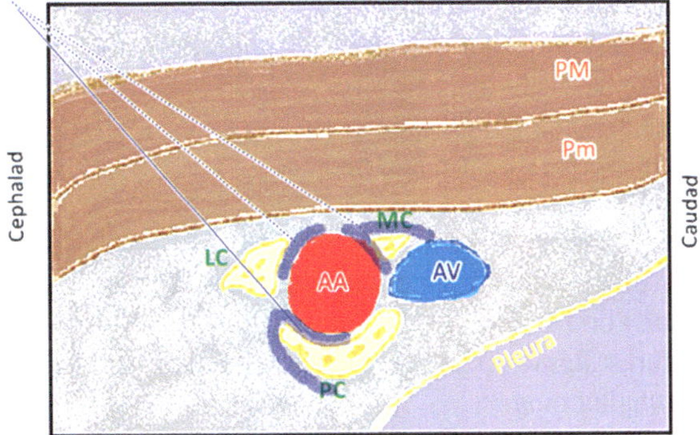

Fig. 2.11 Anatomical basis of infraclavicular block: Note the important landmarks. *AA* axillary artery, *AV* axillary vein, *PM* pectoralis major muscle, *Pm* pectoralis minor muscle, *LC* lateral cord, *MC* medial cord, *PC* posterior cord of the brachial plexus. The blue line represents the needle entry and the dotted lines needle redirections. LA should be spread all around the axillary artery (blue coloured area) for a successful block

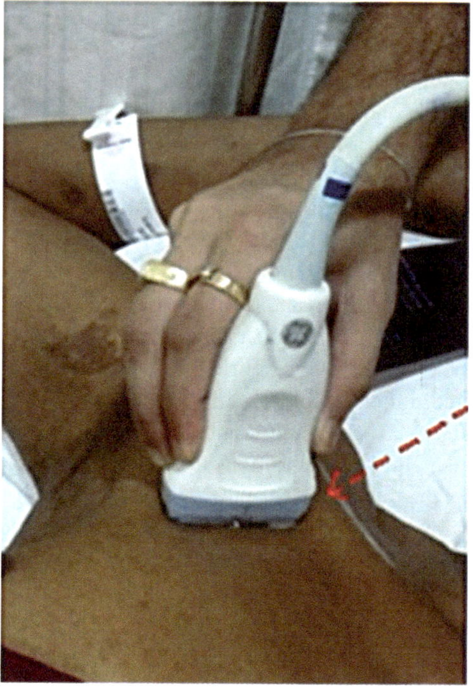

Fig. 2.12 Patient and ultrasound probe position for the infraclavicular block. The red arrow represents the needle entry point and direction

the artery. Nerve becomes prominent within the hypoechoic background of LA. Inject the entire 25–30 ml. If proper distribution of LA could not be achieved, then target the lateral and medial cords separately.

- Bring out the needle and redirect towards lateral and medial cords. Be cautious while blocking the medial cord as it lies between artery and vein and a good plane is always not appreciated for safe needle passage.
- Intermittent aspiration and injection of small aliquots of LA while monitoring the injection pressure if possible (Figs. 2.12 and 2.13).

Indications

Surgery of the arm, elbow, forearm and hand

Blockmate Pearls

- Infraclavicular block is ideal for continuous catheter technique as the pectoral muscles provide good anchorage.
- The area of interest lies deep and requires steep needle insertion. needle visualisation may be challenging.
- There is limited space between clavicle and ultrasound transducer for needle insertion.
- Pneumothorax may happen if pleura is not properly visualised and identified during needling.

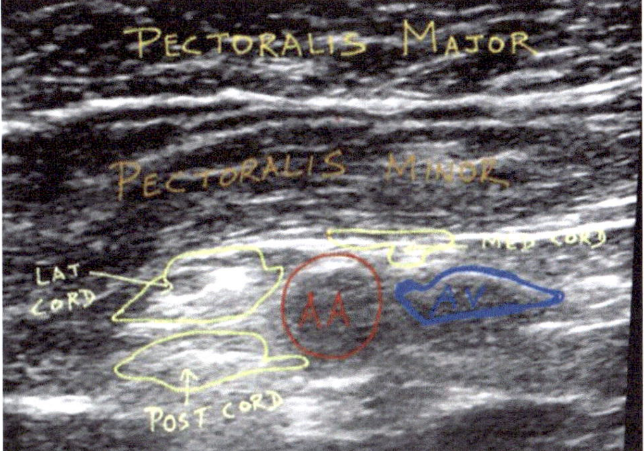

Fig. 2.13 Infra-clavicular block sonoanatomy

- Phrenic nerve palsy, though less than supraclavicular or interscalene, may happen. AN accurate block with low LA volume reduces the risk of phrenic involvement.

2.2.4 The Costoclavicular Block

The costoclavicular block (CCB) is a variant of the infraclavicular block. In contrast to the block at the lateral infraclavicular fossa where the cords are located deep and separated from each other, here the anatomical location of the cords is consistent and clustered together lateral to the axillary artery. Hence a single injection of LA would suffice.

Position The patient lies supine with the ipsilateral arm abducted and 90 degrees flexed at elbow and head turned away to the opposite side. Care should be taken not to hyperabduct the arm. Rest the arm over a padded arm board. The operator should stand at the head end of the patient with the ultrasound machine kept distal to the arm board directly facing the anaesthesiologist (Fig. 2.14).

Anatomical Landmark Midpoint of clavicle

Sonoanatomy Landmarks

- First part of the axillary artery
- Axillary vein medial to the artery
- Subclavius and pectoralis major muscles (Figs. 2.15 and 2.16)

Technique After positioning the patient and application of sterile dressing and draping ASA standard monitors are attached and intravenous access is obtained. The ultrasound transducer is placed transversely below the midpoint clavicle with

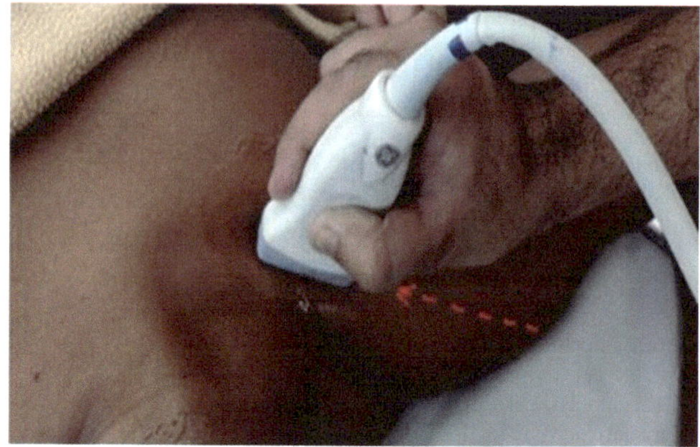

Fig. 2.14 Positioning for Costoclavicular block. The dotted arrow indicates the needle direction

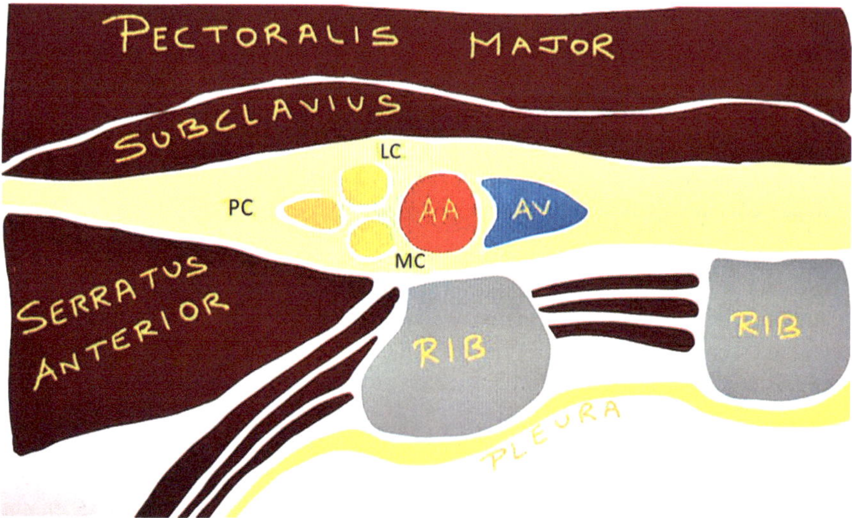

Fig. 2.15 Anatomy of costoclavicular block

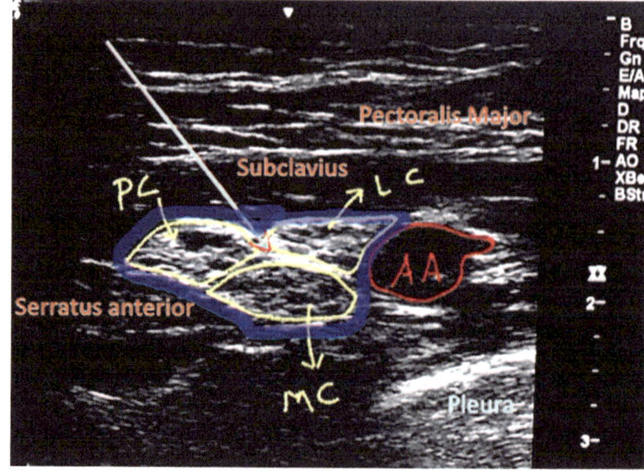

Fig. 2.16 US-guided costoclavicular block: The arrow represents needle trajectory and the LA spread shown as blue colour spread around the cords of brachial plexus: Lateral cord (LC), medial cord (MC) and the posterior cord (PC) are seen clustered together lateral to the axillary artery (AA)

the transducer directed slightly cephalad. Pre injection scanning of the field is done to identify the axillary artery (confirmed with colour doppler showing pulsatile flow), axillary vein (confirmed by compressibility with transducer and with colour doppler showing continuous flow), the cords which are clustered together lateral to the artery and the pleura as a shining hyperechoic line moving with respiration. The needle approaches from the lateral side in plane—full length of the shaft of the needle should be visible all the time.

The needle is brought towards the centre of the cluster and 1–2 ml of 5% dextrose is injected for hydrodissection. Proper placement can be confirmed also by nerve stimulation. Small aliquots of LA are injected and uniform distribution around the cords lateral to the artery is observed. About 20 ml of LA is injected with intermittent aspiration and injection of small aliquots of LA while monitoring the injection pressure.

Indications
Surgery of the arm, elbow, forearm and hand

Blockmate Pearls
- Costoclavicular block is performed with a single injection.
- The onset of action is rapid and predictable.
- Pneumothorax can happen if the pleura is not properly visualised and identified during needling.
- Phrenic nerve palsy may happen but the incidence is lesser than the supraclavicular block.

2.2.5 The Axillary Block

The axillary block is the distal most approach to the brachial plexus. It is also the easiest to perform and the safest. It was the first-ever brachial plexus block described in the days of landmark-based blocks and even with the use of ultrasound, it remains one of the most popular choices among anaesthetists.

Position The patient lies supine with the ipsilateral arm abducted and 90 degrees flexed at the elbow. Care should be taken not to hyperabduct the arm. Rest the arm over a padded arm board. The operator should stand at the head end of the patient with the ultrasound machine kept distal to the arm board directly facing the anaesthesiologist (Fig. 2.17).

Anatomical Landmark Insertion of pectoralis major at the humerus

Ultrasound Anatomy The following are important ultrasound landmarks

- Axillary artery
- Axillary vein medial to the artery
- Conjoint tendon of teres major and latissimus dorsi
- Biceps brachii and coracobrachialis (Figs. 2.18 and 2.19)

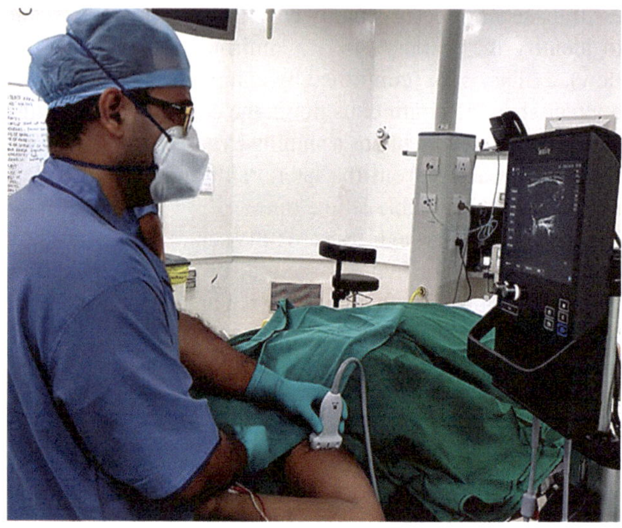

Fig. 2.17 Position for axillary block: Patient lies supine, shoulder abducted at right angle, elbow flexed and arm externally rotated. Note that for a right-sided block, the anaesthetist stands on the head end, keeping the ultrasound monitor at the foot end. For optimum ergonomics, the table height is adjusted to the waist level. The anaesthetists head, the block needle, the US probe and the US monitor all are aligned in a straight line

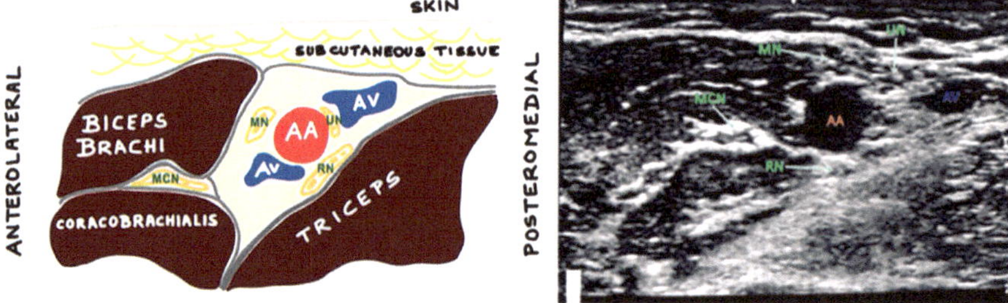

Fig. 2.18 Axillary block anatomy: *AA* axillary artery, *AV* axillary vein

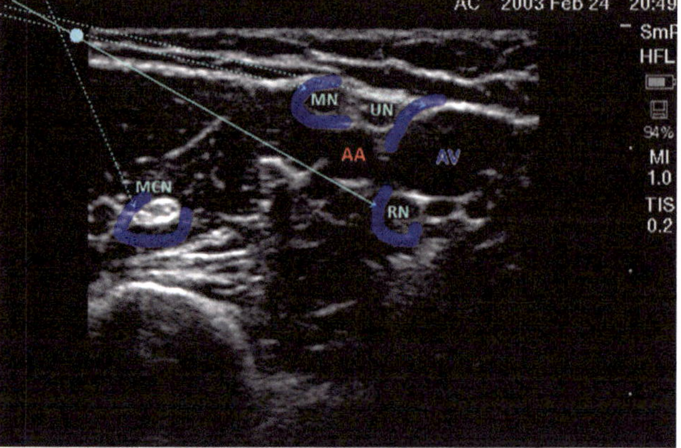

Fig. 2.19 Axillary block technique: The arrow shows the block needle trajectory, the dotted line shows needle redirections required to complete the block along with the block of the musculocutaneous nerve (MCN), which lies lateral to the axillary artery

Block Technique After positioning the patient and application of sterile dressing and draping ASA standard monitors are attached and intravenous access is obtained. Ultrasound transducer is placed transversely just distal to the insertion of the pectoralis major. In the scout scan, the axillary artery needs to be identified and confirmed with colour doppler showing pulsatile flow. The axillary vein should be identified and confirmed by compressibility with UST and with colour doppler showing continuous flow. The conjoint tendon should be identified. The deposition of local anaesthetic just above the tendon and below the axillary artery will almost always block the radial nerve if individual nerve identification becomes difficult. Identify individual nerves—consider the axillary artery as the dial of a clock; median nerve usually lies between 10 o' clock to 1 o' clock position, radial nerve between 7 o' clock to 4 o'clock position and ulnar nerve between artery and vein at 2 o'clock position. The musculocutaneous nerve usually lies separately and anterior/ lateral to the artery between biceps brachii and coracobrachialis muscle and is the brightest structure in the field. The needle should approach from the lateral side in plane. Initially target to bring the needle on the posterior aspect of the axillary artery to block the radial nerve—do not get confused between the nerve and posterior acoustic enhancement. After careful aspiration, inject 1–2 ml of 5% dextrose for hydro dissection and confirm proper placement with nerve stimulation. Thereafter deposit small aliquots of LA and observe for the elevation of the artery. The nerve becomes prominent within the hypoechoic background of LA. Inject 5–7 ml. Bring out the needle and redirect towards the median and ulnar nerves. Deposit 5 ml of LA around each nerve. Be cautious while blocking the ulnar nerve as it lies between artery and vein and a good plane is always not negotiable for safe needle passage. Ulnar nerve often gets blocked while injecting LA for radial nerve block in a U shaped distribution. Before finally taking out the needle, inject 5 ml of LA around the musculocutaneous nerve. Often this nerve may not be separately seen and injecting LA around the median nerve blocks it. It is vital to intermittently aspirate and inject small aliquots of LA while monitoring the injection pressure.

Indications

Surgery of the elbow, forearm and hand

Blockmate Pearls

- Axillary block is the easiest of all brachial plexus blocks to perform. The structures of interest are easily detectable and superficial.
- It is also the safest as there is no risk of pneumothorax or phrenic nerve palsy.
- Inadvertent arterial puncture is easy to control by pressing against the humerus
- Being a distal block of the brachial plexus, it is not suitable for surgeries of the shoulder or upper arm.
- The axillary veins are often compressed by the ultrasound transducer and inadvertent intravascular puncture and local anaesthetic systemic toxicity may happen even with ultrasound.

2.2.6 Distal and Rescue Blocks of the Upper Limb

The supraclavicular block is often called the 'spinal of the upper limb', such as the complete effect it produces. However complete the block may be, be it interscalene or costoclavicular or any other brachial plexus block at any level, even with ultrasound-guided technique, even with the adequately experienced anaesthetist, sometimes there is partial sparing of a particular dermatome/myotome/osteotome. Therefore, before the surgery is allowed to begin or the patient is put under general anaesthesia after administration of the block, it is prudent to check the effect of the block at the dermatome, myotome and osteotome level.

In case there is a sparing, the anaesthetist has two options—(a) to administer general anaesthesia and depend on multimodal analgesia for the intraoperative and postoperative pain and (b) to administer a 'rescue block'.

A 'rescue block' is a distal block of a nerve arising from brachial plexus after the brachial plexus block has been performed but the particular nerve has been spared.

In this chapter, we will enumerate and describe the distal blocks of the upper limb which can also be employed as a rescue block after a partially successful brachial plexus block.

2.2.6.1 Intercostobrachial Nerve Block

Intercostobrachial nerve arises from the second intercostal nerve, which arises from the anterior ramus of the second thoracic spinal nerve (T2) and supplies the inner (medial) aspect of the upper arm. As the origin suggests this nerve is not a component of the brachial plexus and therefore is not blocked by any of the brachial plexus block techniques, and therefore it should not be classified as a 'rescue block'. It has to be blocked separately if the surgery involves the medial aspect of the upper arm or even to cover the pain arising from an upper arm tourniquet.

Technique

The intercostobrachial nerve can be easily blocked by a subcutaneous infiltration of about 5 ml of LA along the axillary crease raising a wheal* of about 2 in. A simple hypodermic needle can be used. Repeated aspiration should be done to avoid inadvertent intravascular injection (Fig. 2.20) (**wheal: raised/ swelling*).

Musculocutaneous Nerve

The musculocutaneous nerve (MCN) innervates the coracobrachialis, biceps brachii and the greater part of the brachialis muscle. Its terminal branch, the lateral cutaneous nerve of the forearm, supplies the sensation of the lateral side of the forearm from the elbow to the wrist. Besides, the musculocutaneous nerve also gives articular branches to the elbow joint and to the humerus. It is usually covered by supraclavicular and infraclavicular brachial plexus blocks. Axillary block tends to spare the MCN.

Block Technique The musculocutaneous nerve usually lies separately and anterior/lateral to the artery between biceps brachii and coracobrachialis muscle and is

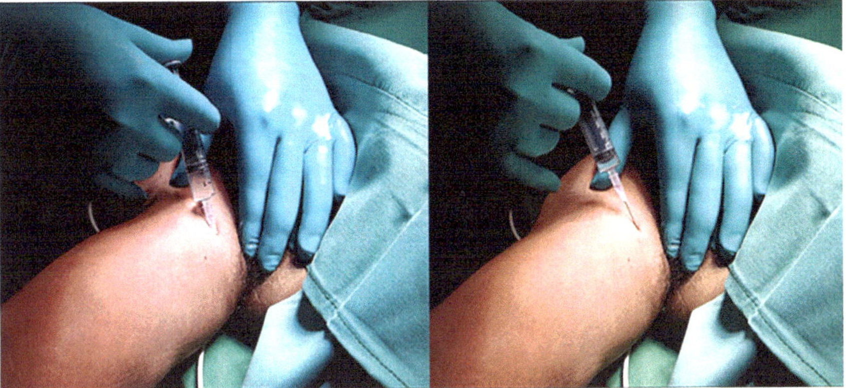

Fig. 2.20 Intercostobrachial nerve block technique

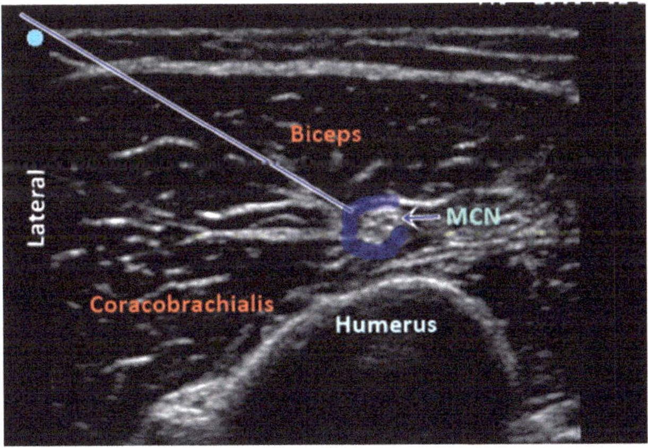

Fig. 2.21 Musculocutaneous nerve block at the mid arm

the brightest structure in the field. In the mid humeral level, the MCN is imaged as a spindle/oval-shaped hyperechoic object 0.5–1 cm above humerus in the plane between biceps brachii and the coracobrachialis. The arm is abducted and UST is placed in the upper 1/3rd of humerus in the midline. The needle is advanced in plane from lateral to medial direction. Five to seven ml LA is usually adequate to block the nerve (Fig. 2.21).

2.2.6.2 Blocks at the Level of Elbow

In the pre-ultrasound era, the nerve blocks at the elbow level were difficult to perform, more time consuming and uncomfortable to the patient. Anatomically the nerves at the elbow are contained in a bony or tight ligamentous surrounding making it more vulnerable for nerve injury. Hence these blocks were not practised widely. Even the ulnar nerve, located superficially, was not blocked due to the risk

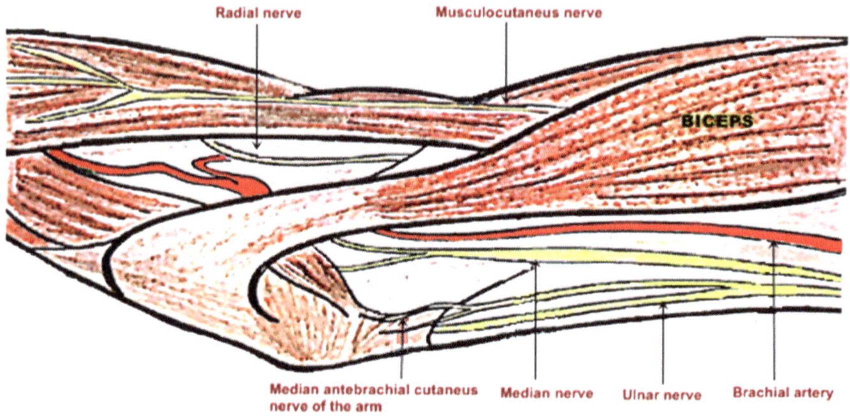

Fig. 2.22 Anatomy of the elbow area

of entrapment neuropathy. With the wide use of the ultrasound, the scenario has changed. The distal nerves can be reliably imaged and blocked now (Fig. 2.22).

The radial, musculocutaneous, median and ulnar nerves can be imaged and blocked in the elbow area.

Median Nerve Block

The median nerve is called the 'eye of the hand'. It supplies the flexor and pronator muscles in the anterior compartment of the forearm except for the flexor carpi ulnaris and part of flexor digitorum profundus (supplied by the ulnar nerve). It also supplies the thenar muscle and lateral two lumbricals in the hand. It lies medially to the brachial artery in the elbow.

Block Technique

The patient lies with the ipsilateral arm resting abducted and supinated on an armrest or hand table. After skin disinfection and sterile draping, the UST is placed 2–3 cm above the cubital crease over the brachial artery. Median nerve lies medially to the brachial artery. 4–5 ml LA is injected around the nerve (Figs. 2.23 and 2.24).

Radial Nerve Block

Radial nerve block is usually performed just above elbow level before its division into superficial and deep branches.

Block Technique

The patient lies with the ipsilateral arm resting abducted and pronated on an armrest or hand table. Alternatively, the arm can be placed on the patient's abdomen with the elbow slightly flexed. After skin disinfection and sterile draping, the UST is placed anterolaterally 3–4 cm above the elbow crease on the groove between the common extensor tendon and biceps muscle. Dual method (US+nerve stimulation) is desirable for confirmation. The UST can be slid up and down the arm for allaying confusion and better imaging. About 5 ml LA is enough to block the nerve (Fig. 2.25).

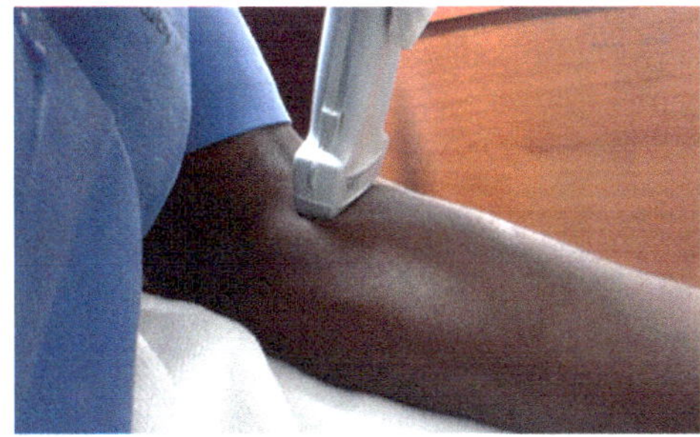

Fig. 2.23 Positioning for median nerve block at the elbow level

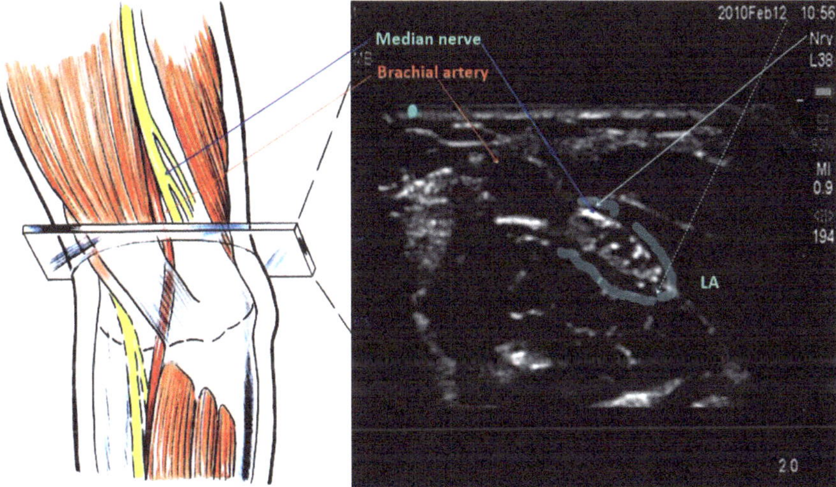

Fig. 2.24 Median nerve block: anatomy and sonoanatomy

Blockmate Pearls

The radial nerve divides just distal to the elbow crease into the superficial (sensory) and deep (motor) branches. These smaller divisions of the radial nerve are more challenging to identify in the forearm; therefore, a single injection above the elbow is favoured because it ensures blockade of both.

Ulnar Nerve Block

The ulnar nerve can be easily identified at the posteromedial aspect of the elbow, 2–3 cm proximal to the crease, as a hyperechoic oval 'honeycomb' like structure immediately underneath the brachial fascia and superficial to the triceps muscle. The ulnar nerve can be traced distally toward the ulnar notch, where it appears as a round hypoechoic structure diving into the bony ulnar sulcus before entering the forearm underneath the flexor carpi ulnaris muscle. Sliding the transducer proximally, the nerve can be traced back to the axilla along the medial aspect of the arm.

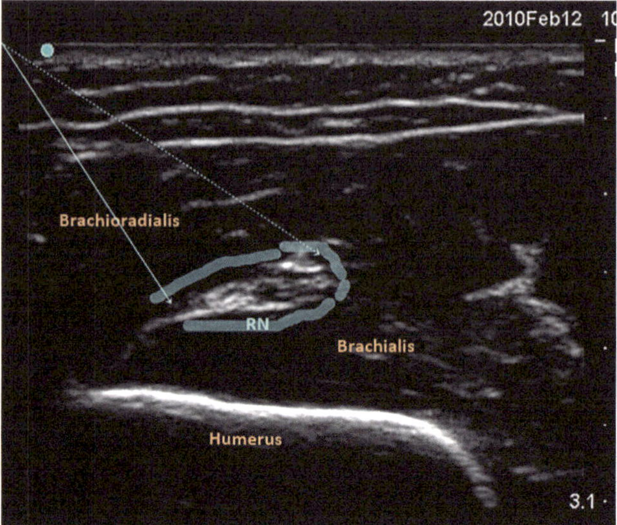

Fig. 2.25 Radial nerve block at the elbow: *RN* radial nerve; the arrow represents the block needle, dotted arrow for redirection of needle

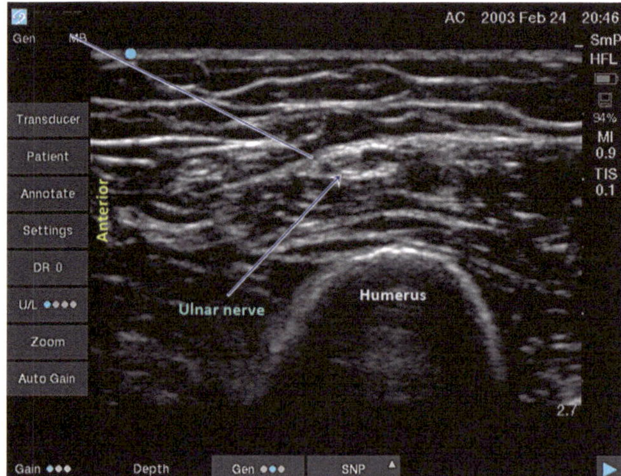

Fig. 2.26 Ulnar nerve block proximal to elbow

Block Technique

The patient lies with the ipsilateral arm resting abducted and flexed at the elbow on an armrest or hand table. After skin disinfection and sterile draping, a high-frequency linear UST is placed transversely 2–3 cm above the cubital crease or the medial epicondyle of humerus on the posteromedial aspect. The ulnar nerve, lying about 1 cm above the humerus can be approached from either side, in plane. About 5 ml LA is usually adequate to block. Using dual technique helps (Fig. 2.26).

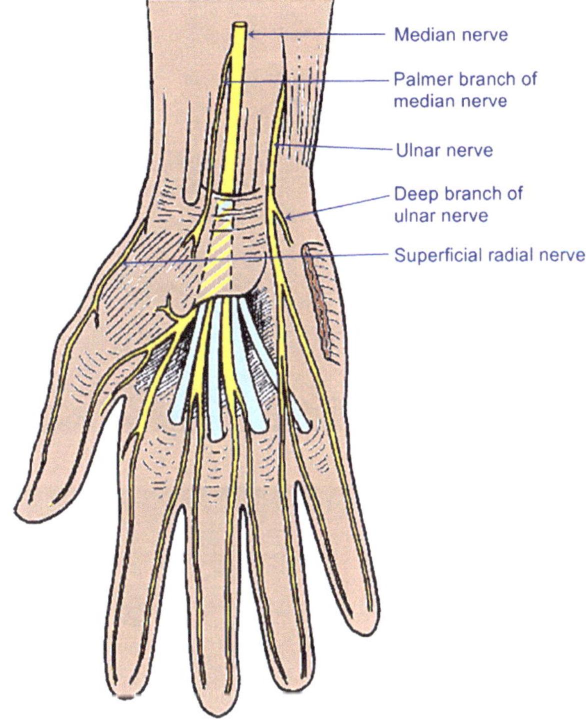

Fig. 2.27 Anatomy of the Wrist

2.2.7 Rescue Blocks at the Level of Wrist

The median nerve innervates the palmar aspect of the first three and a half fingers along with the tip of the dorsal aspect of them. The radial nerve innervates the dorsal aspect of the first three and a half fingers while the ulnar nerve innervates the little finger and ulnar half of the ring finger (Fig. 2.1). All these three nerves can be reliably blocked at the wrist with help of ultrasound [1–7] (Fig. 2.27).

2.2.7.1 Median Nerve Block

The median nerve crosses the elbow medial to the brachial artery and courses toward the wrist deep to the flexor digitorum superficialis in the centre of the forearm. As the muscles taper toward tendons near the wrist, the nerve assumes an increasingly superficial position until it is located beneath the flexor retinaculum in the carpal tunnel with the tendons of the flexor digitorum profundus, flexor digitorum superficialis, and flexor pollicis longus. A linear transducer placed transversely at the level of the wrist crease will reveal a cluster of oval hyperechoic structures, one of which is the median nerve. At this location, it is easy to confuse the tendons for the nerve and vice versa; for this reason, it is recommended to slide the transducer 5–10 cm proximally the volar side of the forearm, to confirm the location of the nerve. The tendons will have disappeared on the image, leaving just muscle and the median nerve, which then can be carefully traced back to the wrist, if desired. In many instances, however, it is much simpler to perform a median nerve block at the mid forearm, where the nerve is easier to recognise.

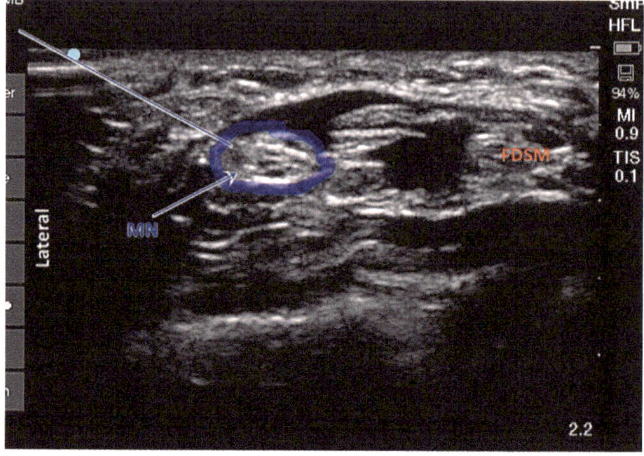

Fig. 2.28 US images of median nerve block at the wrist. *MN* median nerve, *FDSM* flexor digitorum superficialis muscle. Needle approaches from lateral to medial

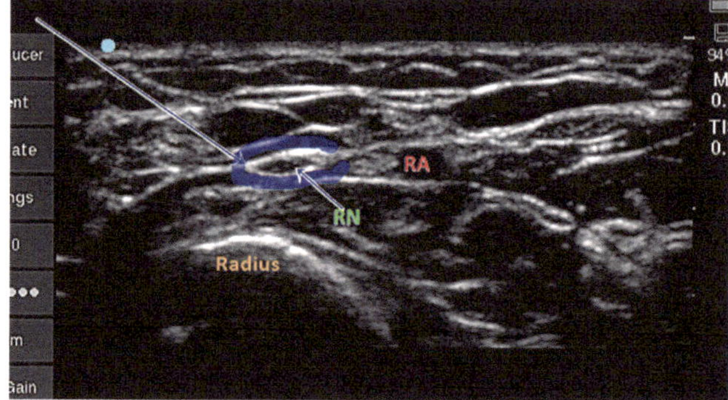

Fig. 2.29 US images of radial nerve block at the wrist. The radial nerve (RN) lies on the radial side of the radial artery (RA). The Block needle enters in plane from the radial side

Block Technique

With the arm in the volar side up position, the skin is disinfected. The median nerve can be blocked either in plane or out-of-plane technique. Three to four ml LA is usually sufficient. Dual technique may be used for nerve confirmation (Fig. 2.28).

2.2.7.2 Radial Nerve Block

The radial nerve lies on the radial side of the radial artery below the flexor retinaculum and medial to the head of the radius.

Block Technique

With the arm in the volar side up position, the skin is disinfected. The radial nerve is approached from the lateral side in plane to avoid injury to the radial artery. Out-of-plane approach can also be employed. Three to four ml LA is usually sufficient. Dual technique may be used for nerve confirmation (Fig. 2.29).

2.2.7.3 Ulnar Nerve Block

The ulnar nerve lies on the ulnar side of the ulnar artery below the flexor carpi ulnaris muscle (FCUM) and lateral to the ulna.

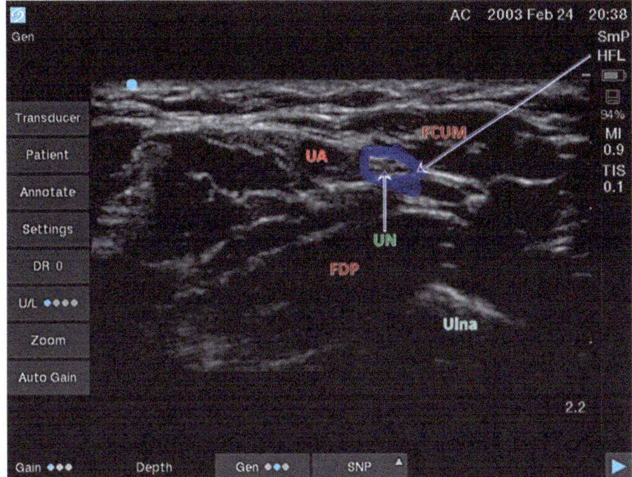

Fig. 2.30 US images of ulnar nerve (UN) block at the wrist. UN lies on the ulnar side of the ulnar artery (UA). Block needle enters from the ulnar side in plane. *FDP* Flexor digitorum profundus, *FCUM* Flexor carpi ulnaris muscle

Block Technique

With the arm in the volar side up position, the skin is disinfected. Ulnar nerve is approached from the medial side in plane to avoid injury to the ulnar artery. LA is deposited between the FCUM and flexor digitorum profundus around the ulnar nerve. Three to four ml LA is usually sufficient. Dual technique may be used for nerve confirmation (Fig. 2.30).

Blockmate Pearls

- The wrist block is an effective method to provide anaesthesia of the hand and fingers without the arm immobility that occurs with more proximal brachial plexus blocks.
- The wrist is a 'tightly packed' area that is bounded on three sides by bones. For this reason, a US-guided 'wrist' block is often performed 5–10 cm proximally to the wrist crease, where there is more room to manoeuvre.
- In addition to providing anaesthesia and analgesia, wrist blocks using botulinum toxin to treat hyperhidrosis have been described.

2.2.8 Regional Anaesthesia for Shoulder Surgery

Regional anaesthesia for shoulder surgery can be achieved in isolation as the primary anaesthetic or in combinations with general anaesthesia for effective postoperative analgesia.

One must remember the anatomy of the shoulder, its dermatome, myotome and osteotome distribution (Figs. 2.1, 2.2, 2.3, and 2.4). The cutaneous innervation of the shoulder and the surrounding area of neck and chest wall is by the supraclavicular nerve (C3-4), which is derived from the superficial cervical plexus, the muscles are supplied mostly by branches of the posterior cord of brachial plexus, while the bones are innervated by the nerve to subclavius, the suprascapular nerves, axillary nerve and a small area at the upper end of the humerus by the radial nerve (Table 2.2).

Three main regimes of administering regional anaesthesia for shoulder surgeries are interscalene nerve block that includes the supraclavicular nerve block, combination of peri-clavicular nerve blocks+ selective supraclavicular nerve block or by local anaesthetic infiltration techniques provided during open surgeries.

A clear discussion of the operative surgery technique will help in determining the extent of sensory nerve blockade. The use of posterior shoulder trocar can result in the need for administration of rescue analgesics and might not be covered in most of the pure regional anaesthetic approaches. Manipulation of frozen shoulder requires very good depth of regional anaesthetic and motor blockade and careful patient selection for the success of the technique.

Table 2.2 Innervation of the shoulder

Area	Nerves	Blocks
Skin	Supraclavicular (C3-4)	Superficial cervical plexus block, skin infiltration over middle third of clavicle
Muscles		
Pectoralis major	Lateral (C5-7) and medial pectoral nerves (C8-T1), branch of the lateral and medial cord of the brachial plexus respectively	Brachial plexus block, supraclavicular/perivascular infraclavicular approaches block the pectoral nerves better than interscalene approach
Pectoralis minor		
Subclavius	Nerve to subclavius (C5-6) from the upper trunk of brachial plexus	Interscalene block
Serratus anterior	Long thoracic nerve (C5-7)	Usually not required. An upper trunk block usually covers long thoracic nerve
Latissimus dorsi	Thoracodorsal nerve	Perivascular brachial plexus block
Deltoid	Axillary nerve (C5-6)	Interscalene block
Supraspinatus	Suprascapular nerve (C4-6)	Interscalene block, upper trunk block
Infraspinatus	Suprascapular nerve (C4-6)	
Teres major	Lower subscapular nerve (C6-7)	Interscalene block, upper trunk block
Teres minor	Axillary nerve (C5-6)	Brachial plexus block
Subscapularis	Upper and lower subscapular nerves (C5-7)	Interscalene block, upper trunk block
Bone/periosteum		
Scapula: anterior surface	Subscapular nerve (C5-7)	Interscalene block, upper trunk block
Scapula: posterior surface, along with the posterior surface of the upper end of the humerus	Suprascapular nerve (C4-6)	
Clavicle	Nerve to subclavius (C5-6)	Brachial plexus block
Humerus-anterior aspect	Axillary nerve (C5-6)	Brachial plexus block

The use of continuous interscalene catheter might be a necessity for effective postoperative analgesia and need to be administered preoperatively with appropriate fixation of catheter away from the field of surgery. Displacement and dislodgement of the catheter are known to be high and require meticulous attention to the technique, needle to catheter exchange, fixation, water-resistant adhesive tape quality, and careful removal of surgical drapes at the end of the operation. Both in plane and out-of-plane catheter placements are known to have similar effects.

2.2.9 Superficial Cervical Plexus Block

The superficial cervical plexus (SCP) lies beneath the lateral border of the sternocleidomastoid muscle (SCM) at the mid length of the muscle. Its position usually corresponds with the point where the external jugular vein crosses the SCM. It gives branches that innervate the head and neck area and the anterior chest wall, extending up to the second rib. It can be easily blocked by the use of ultrasound.

Position Patient lies supine with the head turned to the other side (Fig. 2.31).

Technique With aseptic precautions, the ultrasound transducer (UST) is placed transversely on the neck at the level of the cricoid cartilage and major landmarks such as the common carotid artery and the internal jugular vein (IJV) are identified. SCM is identified as the flat muscle above the IJV. Moving further laterally the lateral border of SCM is identified. Superficial cervical plexus can be identified at this point as 'honeycomb' appearing structures, 2–3 in number inferior to the lateral edge of the SCM. The block needle enters in plane, lateral to medial and the needle is placed between the SCM and the prevertebral fascia. Needle location is confirmed using hydrodissection. Five to seven ml LA is usually sufficient to block the SCP.

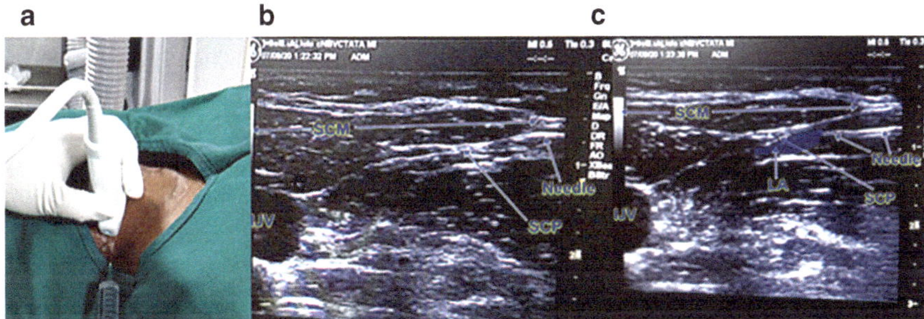

Fig. 2.31 Superficial cervical plexus block: Note the patient lies supine with the head turned to the opposite side (**a**) while the needle is inserted from lateral to medial in plane. A standard hypodermic needle is usually sufficient for this block. Important landmarks in the sonoanatomy (**b**) are the internal jugular vein (IJV) and the sternocleidomastoid muscle (SCM). The needle is placed in plane underneath the lateral border of SCM. Superficial cervical plexus (SCP) can be seen as honeycomb appearing structure beneath the lateral edge of the SCM. Hydrodissection is performed to confirm needle location (**c**) and local anaesthetic (LA) injected to establish the block

Indications

- Shoulder surgery, in conjunction with perivascular brachial plexus block
- Frontal neck surgeries such as thyroidectomy, carotid endarterectomy, etc.

Blockmate Pearls

- The ultrasound-guided superficial cervical plexus block is also called the intermediate cervical plexus block.

2.2.10 Stellate Ganglion Block

The stellate ganglion is formed by the fusion of the inferior cervical ganglion with the first thoracic ganglion. It lies anterior to the transverse process of the seventh cervical vertebra and the neck of the first rib, posteromedial to the apical pleura. It relays the sympathetic outflow to the upper limb and the cardiac plexus.

Indication for Block

Stellate ganglion block (SGB) is useful for diagnosis or treatment of circulation problems or nerve injuries of the upper limb, including:

- Reflex sympathetic dystrophy
- Causalgia
- Complex Regional Pain Syndrome type I or II
- Herpes zoster infection (or 'shingles') affecting the head, neck, arm or upper chest
- Phantom limb pain

It is also useful in treating refractory supraventricular tachycardia.

It has been shown useful in treating post-traumatic stress disorder as it can reduce dysfunctional sympathetic tone, hyperarousal state and inability to relax.

Technique

Patient lies supine, head turned towards the opposite side. Classically SGB has been performed in a landmark-based technique, often aided by fluoroscopy. The technique involves palpation of the carotid tubercle, i.e. the transverse process of the sixth cervical vertebra (C6). The carotid artery and the SCM are retracted laterally with the palpating index finger and the block needle enters perpendicularly to contact the carotid tubercle. After careful aspiration 7 ml LA is injected below the prevertebral fascia and above the longus colli muscle. Fluoroscopy can be used to rule out intramuscular (dye does not spread) and intravascular (dye washes out as soon as injected) placement of the needle. Injected at the right location, the dye spreads along the plane of the cervical sympathetic chain between the prevertebral fascia and the longus colli muscle.

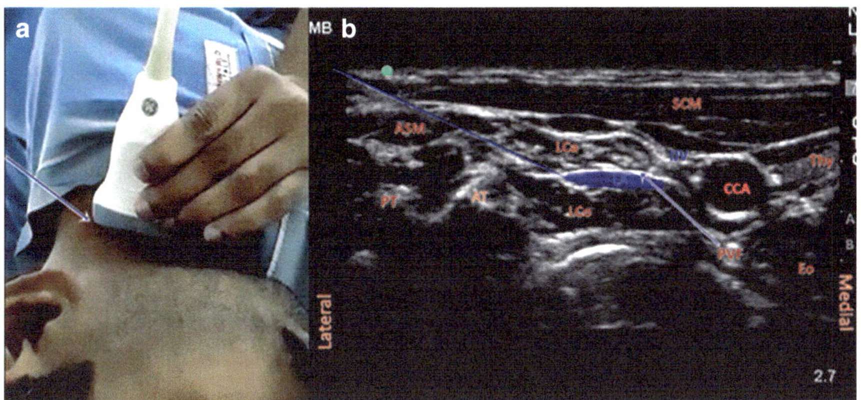

Fig. 2.32 Stellate ganglion block in the lateral approach: (**a**) Patient position, (**b**) US image of the block—sonoanatomy. Arrow represents the needle trajectory. *AT* anterior tubercle, *PT* posterior tubercle, *ASM* anterior scalene muscle, *LCa* longus capitis muscle, *LCo* longus colli muscle, *SCM* sternocleidomastoid muscle, *LA* local anaesthetic, *PVF* prevertebral fascia, *CCA* common carotid artery, *Thy* thyroid, *Eo* oesophagus. Note the internal jugular vein (IJV) is compressed with the ultrasound probe

The ultrasound-guided technique has made the block safer as it has reduced inadvertent vascular or pleural injury. Instead of the palpating finger a high-frequency linear probe is placed transversely over the C6 and pressed to move the carotid artery laterally and the trachea medially. A 25G needle is inserted in plane from medial to lateral direction targeting the middle of the longus colli muscle. The needle is advanced till it pierces the prevertebral fascia and lies just above the longus colli muscle. Hydro dissection is done to confirm needle location. 10 ml LA is injected in small aliquots with repeated aspirations.

Alternatively, in the lateral approach, the patient lies lateral with the neck extended and the head supported on a pillow (Fig. 2.32). The high-frequency UST is held transversely at the level of the sixth cervical vertebra. Important landmarks are imaged and the probe is placed between the transverse process of the C6 laterally and the common carotid artery medially. The needle enters in plane from lateral to medial till it pierces the prevertebral fascia covering the longus colli muscle and 10 ml LA is deposited in small aliquots between the fascia and the muscle after careful aspiration [8].

The lateral approach is safer as it avoids injury to the vertebral artery, thyroid gland, vagus nerve, thoracic duct and the oesophagus. The patient is also more comfortable as pressure on the trachea is avoided.

Acknowledgement Dr. Amit Dikshit for rescue block images and Dr. Rajendra Sahoo for Stellate ganglion block images.

References

1. Olea E, Fondarella A, Sánchez C, Iriarte I, Almeida MV, Martínez de Salinas A. Bloqueo de los nervios periféricos a nivel de la muñeca guiado por ecografía para el tratamiento de la hiperhidrosis idiopática palmar con toxina botulínica [Ultrasound-guided peripheral nerve block at wrist level for the treatment of idiopathic palmar hyperhidrosis with botulinum toxin]. Rev Esp Anestesiol Reanim. 2013;60:571–5.
2. Bajaj S, Pattamapaspong N, Middleton W, Teefey S. Ultrasound of the hand and wrist. J Hand Surg Am. 2009;34:759–60.
3. Heinemeyer O, Reimers CD. Ultrasound of radial, ulnar, median and sciatic nerves in healthy subjects and patients with hereditary motor and sensory neuropathies. Ultrasound Med Biol. 1999;25:481–5.
4. Kiely PD, O'Farrell D, Riordan J, Harmon D. The use of ultrasound-guided hematoma blocks in wrist fractures. J Clin Anesth. 2009;21:540–2.
5. Liebmann O, Price D, Mills C, et al. Feasibility of forearm ultrasonography guided nerve blocks of the radial, ulnar, and median nerves for hand procedures in the emergency department. Ann Emerg Med. 2006;48:558–62.
6. Macaire P, Singelyn F, Narchi P, Paqueron X. Ultrasound- or nerve stimulation guided wrist blocks for carpal tunnel release: a randomized prospective comparative study. Reg Anesth Pain Med. 2008;33:363–8.
7. McCartney CJL, Xu D, Constantinescu C, et al. Ultrasound examination of peripheral nerves in the forearm. Reg Anesth Pain Med. 2007;32:434–9.
8. Peng PW, Narouze S. Ultrasound-guided interventional procedures in pain medicine: a review of anatomy, sonoanatomy, and procedures: Part I: Nonaxial structures. Reg Anesth Pain Med. 2009;34:458–74.

Lower Extremity Nerve Blocks

3

Sudhakar Subramani and Sangini Punia

3.1 Introduction

Many techniques for lower extremity blocks have been described over time to facilitate surgery on the lower extremity as well as improve postoperative analgesia. Lower extremity nerve blocks can play an important role in preventing the development of chronic pain in patients requiring limb amputation [1]. In addition, regional anesthesia for the lower extremity has been proven to be extremely safe and provides improved pain control when used as a part of a well-designed multimodal anesthetic technique [2]. In resource-poor settings, as well as in cases of complex patients with multiple severe comorbidities, regional anesthesia techniques can help decrease/eliminate complications of endotracheal intubation and the cardiac depressant effects of general anesthesia. In this chapter we will discuss the anatomy and innervation of the lower extremity followed by the common lower extremity nerve blocks, progressing from proximal to distal (Table 3.1).

3.2 Anatomy and Innervation of Lower Extremity

The lower extremity is supplied by the lumbar plexus which innervates the anterior aspect, and the sacral plexus which innervates mostly the posterior aspects. We will briefly describe the salient nerves to facilitate a deeper understanding of nerve blocks in the lower extremity.

S. Subramani (✉) · S. Punia
Department of Anesthesia, University of Iowa, Iowa City, IA, USA
e-mail: Sudhakar-subramani@uiowa.edu; Sangini-punia@uiowa.edu

A. Chakraborty (ed.), *Blockmate*, https://doi.org/10.1007/978-981-15-9202-7_3

Table 3.1 Anatomic location of various nerve blocks for lower extremity

Paraspinal region	Lumbar plexus	Analgesia for anterior and medial thigh, anterior and medial leg, knee
Hip	Sciatic nerve • Subgluteal approach • Parasacral approach • Classical approach • Anterior approach	Analgesia for posterior thigh, leg, and majority of foot
	Femoral nerve	Analgesia for anterior thigh, knee
	Three-in-one block/Fascia Iliaca block • Femoral, obturator, and lateral femoral cutaneous nerve	Analgesia for anterior, medial, and lateral thigh, as well as knee
Thigh	Sciatic nerve • Popliteal approach	Analgesia for knee, lower leg, and foot
	Saphenous nerve • Adductor canal	Analgesia for medial knee and medial leg and foot
Leg	Saphenous nerve	Analgesia for medial leg and foot
Foot	Ankle block	Analgesia for forefoot and toes

3.2.1 Lumbar Plexus

The lumbar plexus originates from the anterior rami of L1–L4 spinal nerves and lies within the psoas muscle. The plexus forms various peripheral nerves that run down the posterior abdominal wall toward their target structures. Relevant branches of the lumbar plexus that innervate the lower extremity include the lateral Femoral cutaneous Nerve of Thigh, Femoral Nerve, and Obturator nerve. In addition, the lumbar plexus also forms the Iliohypogastric nerve (sensory to posterolateral gluteal skin), the ilioinguinal nerve (sensory to the skin over the superior anteromedial aspect of thigh), and the genitofemoral nerve (the femoral branch of which innervates the superior aspect of the anterior thigh as shown in Fig. 3.1).

Lateral Femoral Cutaneous Nerve of Thigh—Nerve Roots L2 and 3
Enters from the lateral aspect of the inguinal ligament and is a purely sensory nerve. It provides sensation to the anterior and lateral aspects of the thigh from the inguinal ligament down to the knee. This nerve may be blocked individually or with a supra-inguinal fascia iliaca block (3-in-1 block) to facilitate analgesia in patients with hip fractures or undergoing hip surgery.

Obturator Nerve—Nerve Roots L2–L4
This nerve is a mixed sensory and motor nerve. It is formed by receiving contributions from the L2, 3, and 4 nerve roots. Once formed, it descends straight down within the body of the psoas muscle and emerges from it at the medial border. The nerve travels close to the iliac vessels along the posterior pelvis toward the obturator foramen of the ilium. At the obturator foramen, the obturator nerve enters the thigh

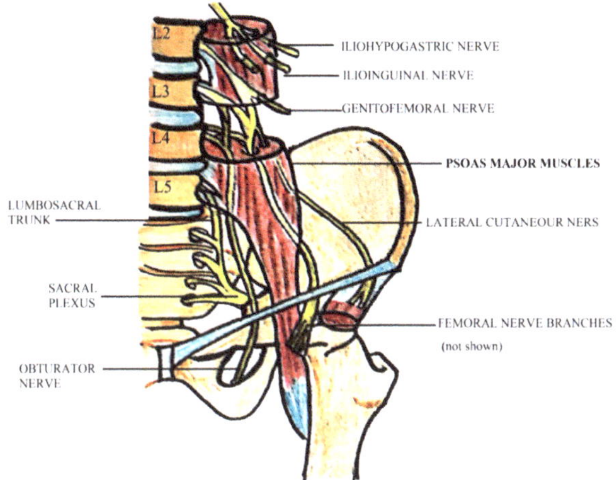

Fig. 3.1 Lumbar plexus formation and course within the pelvis

and divides into an anterior and posterior branch [3]. The obturator nerve provides sensation to the medial thigh, and motor supply to the majority of muscles in the medial thigh—obturator externus, pectineus, adductor longus, adductor brevis, adductor magnus, and gracilis. This nerve may be blocked individually, however more commonly blocked in combination with the Femoral and Lateral Cutaneous Nerve of thigh while performing a 3-in-1 block for hip surgery/trauma.

Femoral Nerve—Nerve Roots L2–L4

The femoral nerve supplies the skin of the anterior thigh and it is a mixed nerve. A branch of the femoral nerve, the saphenous nerve supplies a strip of skin over the medial aspect of the lower leg. The motor supply of the Femoral nerve extends to the muscles in the front of the thigh—pectineus, Sartorius, and quadratus femoris. In the pelvis, the femoral nerve also supplies the iliacus muscle. This nerve can be blocked individually (most common) or with the 3-in-1 block (Fig. 3.2).

3.2.2 Sacral Plexus

The sacral plexus is formed by the anterior rami of S1–S4 nerve roots, with contribution from the L4 and L5 roots. It is located anterior to the pyriformis muscle and supplies the posterior aspect of the thigh as well as the majority of the leg and foot. The nerve roots combine to form various cords that descend down the pelvis and ultimately form the five major peripheral nerves of the sacral plexus. Figure 3.3 depicted the formation of the sacral plexus within the pelvis; and Fig. 3.4 showed the course of the nerves arising from the sacral plexus within the lower extremity.

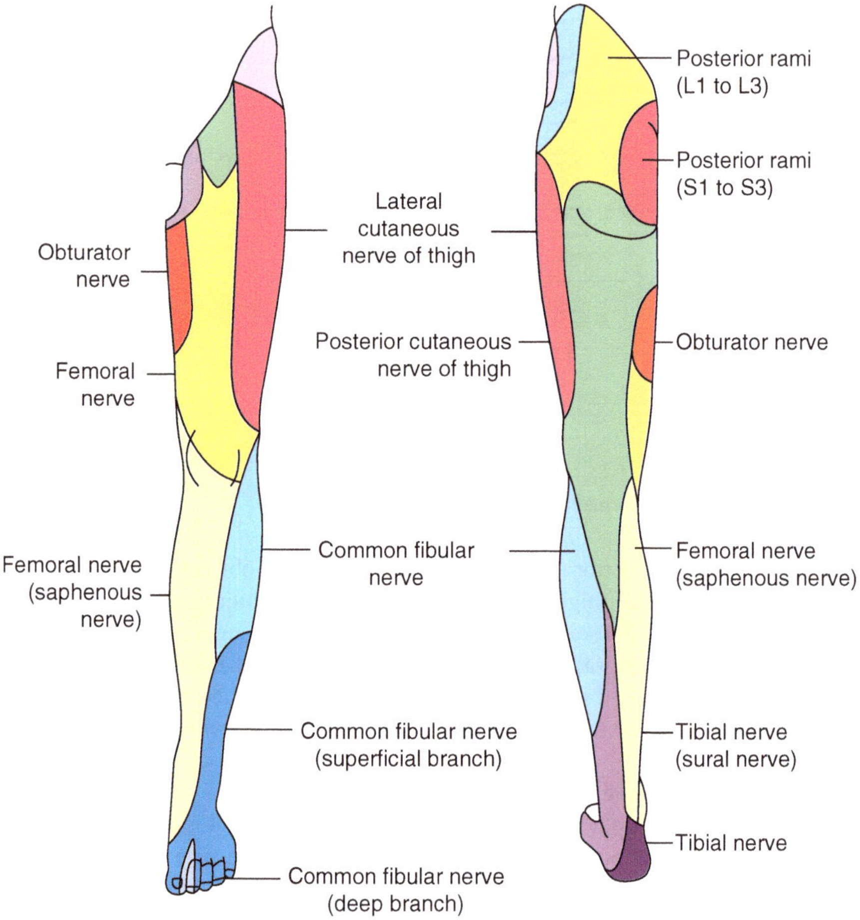

Fig. 3.2 Sensory distribution of the lower extremity

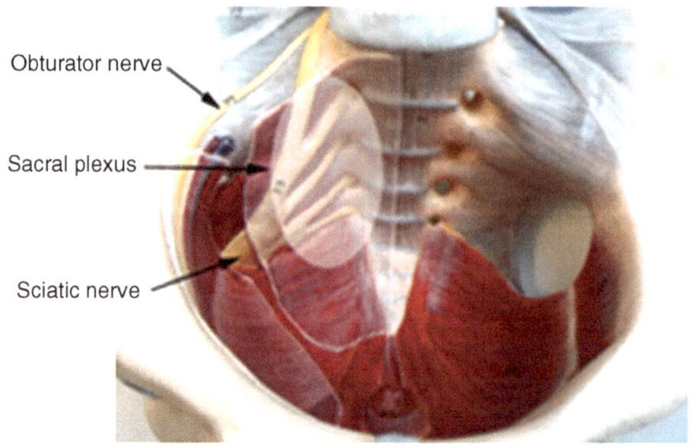

Fig. 3.3 Formation of the sacral plexus (http://www.dontbeasalmon.net/archives/2010/05/anatomy-the-lum.html)

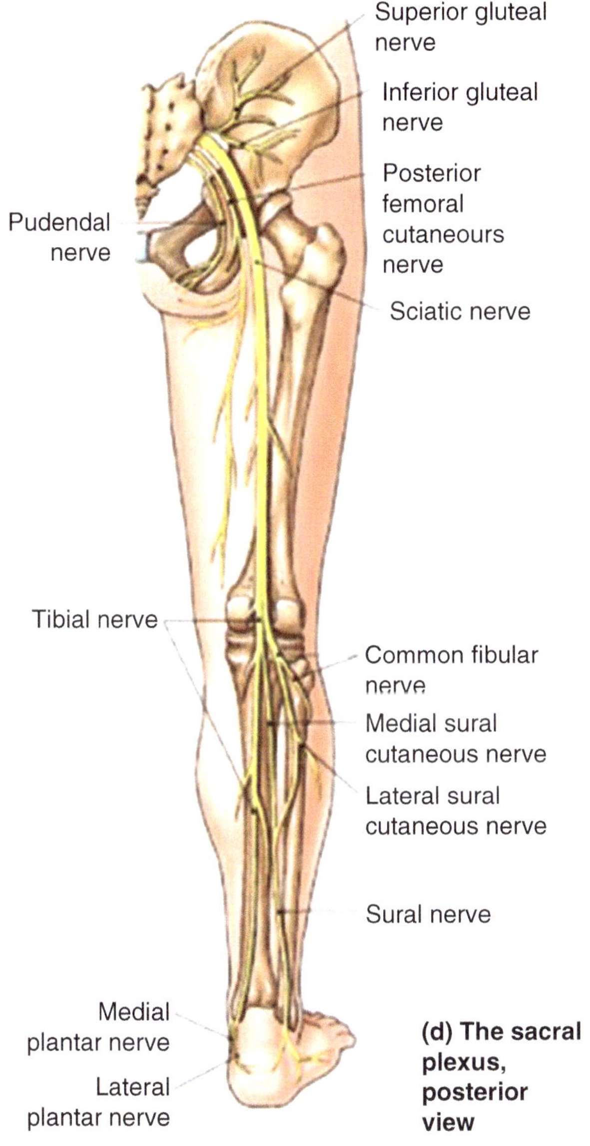

Fig. 3.4 Innervation of the lower extremity arising from the sacral plexus

Superior Gluteal Nerve—Nerve Roots L4, L5, S1

Leaves the pelvis at the greater sciatic foramen and is accompanied by the artery and vein of the same name. It innervates the gluteus minimus, gluteus medius, and tensor fascia lata.

Inferior Gluteal Nerve—Nerve Roots L5, S1, S2

This nerve also exits the pelvis at the greater sciatic foramen and runs inferiorly to the superior gluteal nerve. It supplies the gluteus maximus.

Sciatic Nerve—Nerve Roots L4, L5, S1, S2, S3

This nerve provides sensory and motor innervation to a large part of the posterior thigh, leg, and foot. It originates from the ventral rami of L4–S3 spinal nerves which converge to form a single nerve close to the vertebral bodies. The sciatic nerve then exits the pelvis through the greater sciatic foramen. It descends into the posterior compartment of the thigh deep to the biceps femoris muscles, superficial to adductor magnus and lateral to the semitendinosus and semimembranosus. Just before entering the popliteal fossa, it divides into its two main branches—Tibial Nerve and Common Peroneal nerve [4]. Tibial Nerve provides sensation to the posterolateral leg, lateral border of the foot, and sole of the foot. Its motor supply extends to the muscles in the back of the thigh (except the short head of biceps femoris). It innervates all the muscles in the back of the leg and the sole of the foot. Figure 3.5 shows the sensory distribution of the foot—this becomes especially relevant when performing ankle block for foot surgery. Common Peroneal Nerve provides sensation to the skin over the lateral aspect of the leg and the dorsum of the foot. It provides motor supply to the short head of biceps femoris, all muscles in the anterior and lateral compartments of the leg, as well as extensor digitorum brevis in the foot.

There is considerable variation in the division of the sciatic nerve into its two main branches. One study that examined 140 cadaveric lower extremities found that the sciatic nerve divided within the popliteal fossa in 58% of the specimens, at the upper 1/3rd of thigh in 31% of specimens. The remaining specimens ~9% had a higher bifurcation close to the pyriformis muscle in the gluteal region [5]. This anatomical variation may influence clinical decision making by both surgeons and

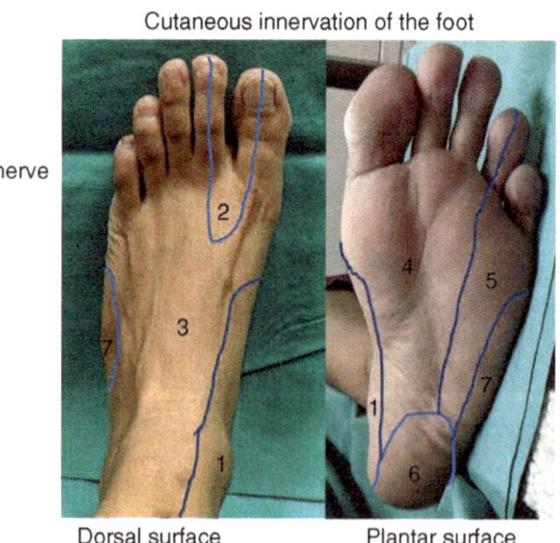

Fig. 3.5 Sensory innervation of the ankle and foot

anesthesiologists in case of sciatic nerve injury during surgery or trauma. In addition, recognition of anatomical variations is important when making a decision regarding regional anesthesia and choosing the appropriate peripheral nerve block technique.

Posterior Femoral Cutaneous Nerve—Nerve Roots S1–S3
Also leaves the pelvis at the greater sciatic foramen and descends deep to the gluteus maximus. Innervates skin on the perineum, as well as the skin over the posterior surface of thigh and leg.

OTHER NERVES arising from sacral plexus—Most of these small nerves directly innervate muscles in the lower extremity. These are nerve to obturator internus, nerve to pyriformis, and nerve to quadratus femoris. A sensory nerve, the perforating cutaneous nerve supplies the skin of the inferior gluteal area [6].

3.2.3 Lumbar Plexus Block or Psoas Compartment Block

Indications This is a challenging block to perform as it is difficult to target all the roots of the lumbar plexus and achieve an adequate spread of the injectate. When successful, this block should provide analgesia across all the nerves arising from the lumbar plexus. It is useful for analgesia following femur fractures, hip surgeries, and surgery on the anterior aspect of the thigh and knee. Unfortunately, this block is not sufficient as the sole anesthetic technique as the posterior aspects of the thigh and leg receive a significant contribution from the sacral plexus. This block will produce motor weakness in the region, in addition to the loss of sensation. However, an advantage is that it will cause less sympathectomy compared to spinal anesthetic [7].

Position Lateral decubitus with side to be blocked in the non-dependent position (Fig. 3.6).

Anatomical Technique Important landmarks include the midline (spinous process) and the superior border of the iliac crest. The needle is inserted perpendicular to the skin at 4 cm lateral to the intersection of the above landmarks. A peripheral nerve stimulator should be connected at this time and set to deliver a current >1 mA. As the needle is inserted, the first twitch should correspond to the local twitching of the paravertebral muscles. The needle should be advanced further until a quadriceps twitch on the ipsilateral side is noticed. At this point, the current should be reduced to 0.5–0.8 mA making sure that the stimulation is consistent. Local anesthetic should be injected slowly after aspirating to rule out accidental intravascular placement. About 30–35 mL of local anesthetic is necessary for sufficient injectate spread.

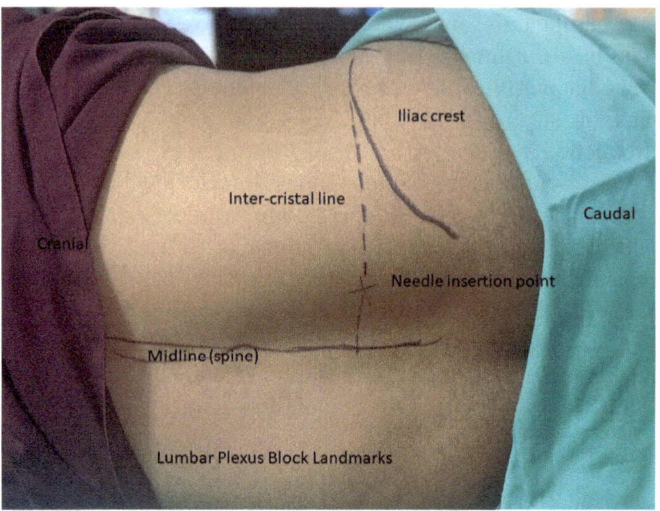

Fig. 3.6 Lateral decubitus position for lumbar plexus block

Ultrasound-Guided Technique The use of ultrasound may reduce the complication rate and improve the accuracy of this block [8], however, due to the deep structures and muscle planes involved sonoanatomy of this block may prove to be challenging. The curved array (low-frequency) transducer should be used for better tissue penetration. The lumbar plexus is not easily identified on sonography, however, in some patients, it appears as a hypoechoic structure within the psoas muscle. Visualization of the plexus may improve upon the injection of a local anesthetic to surround the plexus which will improve its echogenicity.

The patient is positioned in the same way as described for the anatomical technique. The ultrasound probe is placed in a paramedian sagittal plane at the level of L3 and L4 on the side to be blocked. The optimal ultrasound image shows the lumbar "trident" formed by the transverse processes of the lumbar vertebrae (Fig. 3.7). The aim is to guide the needle (inserted from the caudal side of the transducer) into the posterior aspect of the psoas muscle while monitoring for quadriceps twitch similar to the landmark technique. At that point, after negative aspiration, the spread of local anesthetic can be visualized in real time. During and after injection, the plexus may itself become more prominent.

Complications of lumbar plexus block include inadvertent spinal and epidural injection, intravascular injection (ascending lumbar arteries and veins are present in the psoas muscle plane), psoas hematoma, and retroperitoneal hematoma. Hematomas are more common with multiple needle insertions in anticoagulated patients [9].

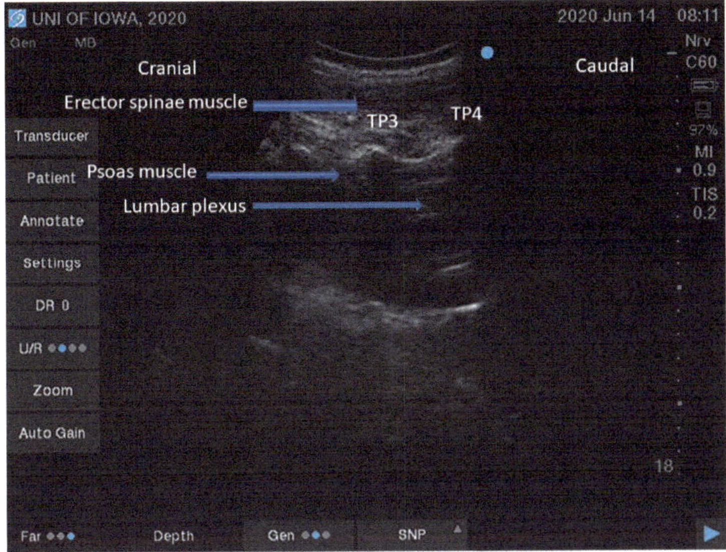

Ultrasonography of Lumbar Plexus demonstrating the 'Lumbar Trident'

Fig. 3.7 Ultrasound imaging of lumbar plexus shows lumbar trident

3.2.3.1 Clinical Implications

For patients who are anticoagulated, or require anticoagulation in the immediate postoperative period, risks of lumbar plexus block may outweigh the benefits. Retroperitoneal hematomas have been reported in the certain patient populations [10]. Compared to spinal anesthesia, the lumbar plexus block produces greater hemodynamic stability, improved ability to ambulate and decreased urinary retention [11, 12]. A randomized, placebo-controlled trial with 50 patients found that ambulatory continuous lumbar plexus block decreased the time to discharge by 38% following hip arthroplasty [12]. However, for intertrochanteric surgery, the combination of femoral block and spinal anesthesia was comparable to lumbar plexus block in terms of analgesia and safety. Overall more effective anesthesia and longer acting analgesia resulted from using the combination of spinal anesthetic and femoral nerve block [13].

3.2.4 Three-in-One Block or Fascia Iliaca Block

Indications Indications are similar to those for Lumbar plexus block—including analgesia for hip, anterior and lateral thigh, and knee surgery. The three nerves blocked in this technique are the femoral nerve, the lateral cutaneous nerve of the thigh, and the obturator nerve. There will be no sciatic coverage with this block. It is less challenging to perform compared to the lumbar plexus block.

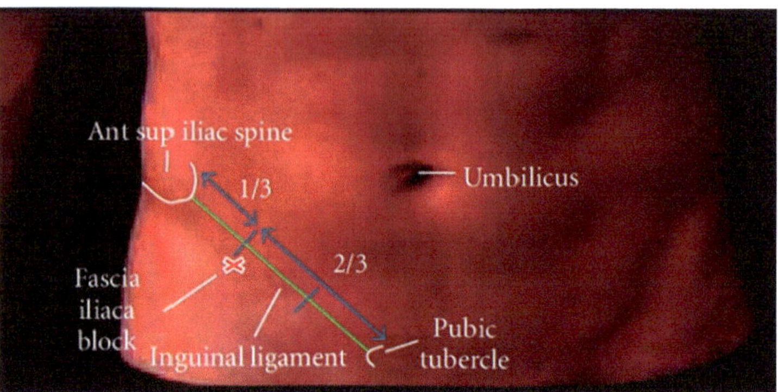

Fig. 3.8 Anatomical landmarks for fascia iliaca nerve block (https://www.hindawi.com/journals/isrn/2011/421505/#copyright)

Position Patient is placed supine with the leg on the side to be blocked extended straight. To facilitate exposure of the groin, slight abduction and/or lateral rotation at the hip may be beneficial. The knee may be flexed to less than 90 degrees for comfort in a "frog leg" position.

Anatomical Technique The goal of fascia iliaca block is to deposit a large volume of local anesthetic within the fascia iliaca compartment, near the femoral nerve. The proximal spread of injectate will then block the lateral cutaneous nerve as well as the obturator nerve; both of which lie within the fascia iliaca compartment during their proximal course. Landmarks for this block are the inguinal ligament, anterior superior iliac spine, and pubic tubercle. A line is drawn connecting the ASIS to the pubic tubercle and then divided into thirds (Fig. 3.8). The needle is inserted at a point 1 cm distal to the junction of the lateral one-third and medial two-thirds of the line. A "pop" or "give" may be felt as the needle penetrates the fascia lata. A second "pop" will be felt after penetrating the fascia iliaca. After negative aspiration, 30–40 mL of local anesthetic can be injected. This is a fascial plane block, thus it's a success depends on the adequate spread of local anesthetic.

Ultrasound-Guided Suprainguinal Technique In this technique, the goal is to target local anesthetic spread to the proximal portions of the three nerves which have not yet emerged out of the fascia iliaca compartment. The patient is positioned similarly to the anatomic technique and a high-frequency (straight) ultrasound probe is placed in a sagittal plane over the ASIS (Fig. 3.9). Sliding the probe medially will reveal a "bow tie" sign (Fig. 3.10) which is easily identified as the muscle fascia converge across the ASIS. The fascia iliaca is identified as deep to the deep circumflex artery. Using an in-plane approach, the needle is inserted from the caudal end of the probe and the tip is positioned beneath the fascia iliaca. An injection is made at this point, with the spread of the injectate cranial to the point where the iliac muscle passes under the abdominal muscle. A similar volume of local anesthetic is necessary with ultrasound-guided technique ~30–40 mL.

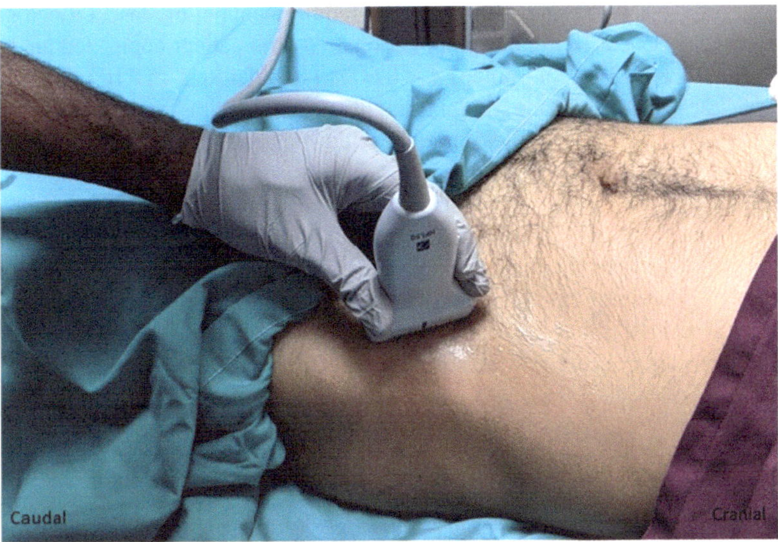

Fig. 3.9 Ultrasound probe positioning for fascia iliaca block

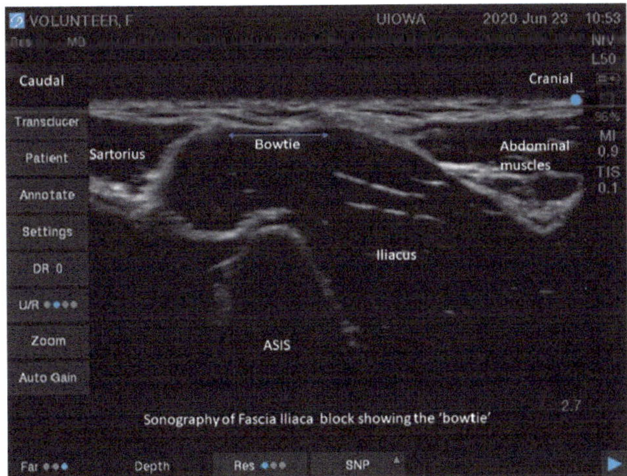

Fig. 3.10 "Bow tie" is seen at the confluence of abdominal musculature and sartorius muscle during ultrasonography for suprainguinal fascia iliaca block

3.2.4.1 Clinical Implications

Fascia iliaca block can be performed in the emergency department for acute relief of pain following a hip fracture. In one study of 106 patients, Fascia iliaca block resulted in better analgesia compared with patient-controlled analgesia. Patients with the fascia iliaca block had lower pain scores at 2, 4, 6, 12, 24, and 48 h, post-surgery ($p = 0.03$). In addition, opioid requirements in the fascia iliaca group were lower (7.35 ± 2.18 mg morphine) compared with patient-controlled analgesia group (65.83 ± 2.13 mg morphine) $p < 0.0001$ [14]. An RCT of 110 patients with femoral neck fracture comparing fascia iliaca block with femoral nerve block showed that Femoral nerve block may provide superior analgesia, however it was clinically insignificant ($p = 0.47$) [15]. As such, further studies and meta-analyses are needed to identify which block is superior and safer for hip analgesia. For knee surgeries like Total knee arthroplasties, one study found no difference in postoperative pain between adductor canal block and femoral nerve block, however quadriceps function was preserved in case of adductor canal block (described later in the chapter). Adductor canal block may be safer in elderly patients prone to falls or ambulatory surgery as muscle weakness is less frequently encountered [16].

3.2.5 Femoral Nerve Block

Indications Analgesia for anterior thigh, anterior hip, and knee procedures. It can also provide analgesia for superficial procedures over the medial aspect of the lower leg (saphenous nerve distribution). Continuous catheter technique can be used to provide analgesia for patients with the femoral shaft or neck fractures with minimal opioids.

Position Patient is positioned similar to the 3-in-1 block as described above.

Anatomical Technique The goal is to inject local anesthetic within the two layers of the fascial iliaca with an infrainguinal approach. Infrainguinally, the femoral sheath contains (from medial-to-lateral) femoral vein, femoral artery, and femoral nerve. The key landmarks to this approach is the inguinal ligament and femoral artery pulsation prominence. The site of needle insertion is slightly inferior to the inguinal crease 1–2 cm lateral to the femoral artery pulsation (Fig. 3.11). The needle is advanced and two "pops" will be felt as the needle traverses the fascia lata and fascia iliaca. A peripheral nerve stimulator should be used to identify a quadriceps twitch/patellar twitch. The needle is optimally positioned when a patellar twitch is obtained between 0.3 and 0.5 mA current. At this point, after negative aspiration, 15–20 mL of local anesthetic is injected.

Ultrasound-Guided Technique This is performed with a high-frequency probe (straight probe) placed parallel to and slightly inferior to the inguinal crease (Fig. 3.12). The Femoral artery and vein and recognized within the femoral sheath (Fig. 3.13). Slight craniocaudal tilting movements of the probe will reveal the femoral nerve as a honeycomb structure present lateral to the femoral vessels. The needle is advanced in an in-plane manner from lateral to medial side with the aim to position the tip within the fascia iliaca but lateral to the femoral nerve. After negative aspiration, 15–20 mL of local anesthetic is injected with visualization of real-time spread around the femoral nerve. Spread laterally to, or immediately posterior to the femoral nerve is adequate for this block and circumferential spread is not essential for success [17].

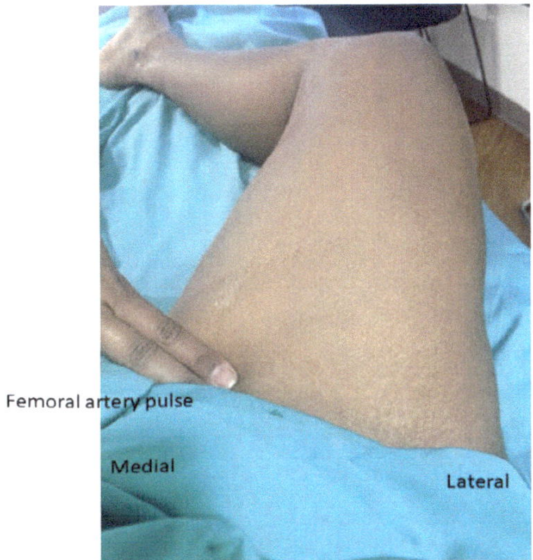

Fig. 3.11 Landmarks for femoral nerve block

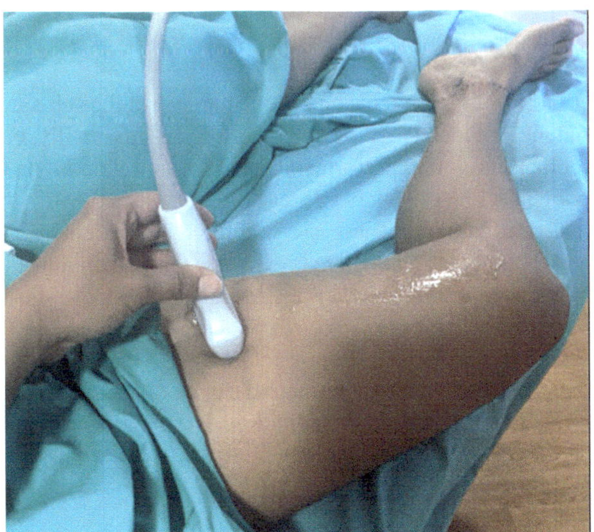

Fig. 3.12 Ultrasound probe position for femoral nerve block

3.2.5.1 Clinical Implications

Femoral nerve block can result in significant weakness with knee extension and may cause falls, especially in the elderly and other at-risk patients. For this reason, it may be somewhat safer to perform an adductor canal block instead (described later in the chapter) [18]. With the adductor canal block, the goal is to inject the local anesthetic distal to the takeoff of the Nerve to vastus medialis, thus preserving quadriceps function. The adductor canal block is essentially a saphenous nerve

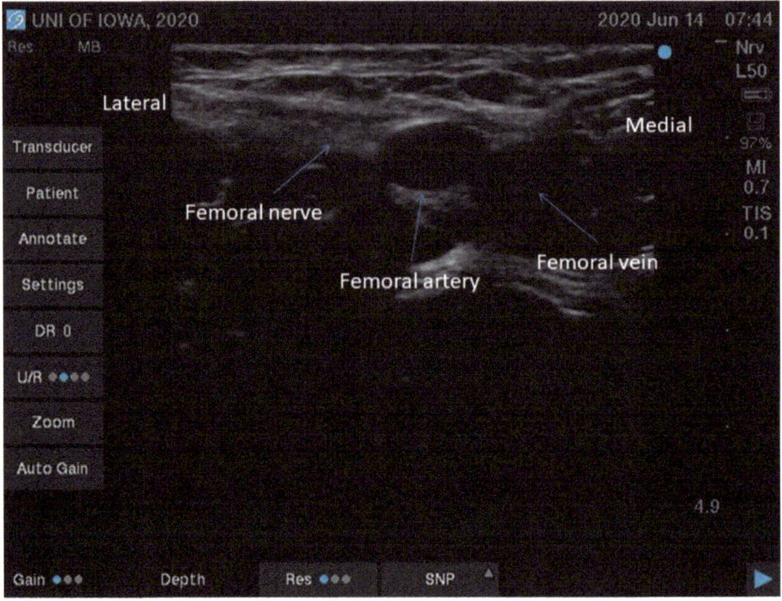

Fig. 3.13 Ultrasound image shows the relationship between femoral nerve and femoral vessels

block, however large volume of local anesthetic injected at the sub-sartorial can still result in a partial motor blockade if the injectate spreads proximally. For this reason, adductor canal blocks are often performed as distal as possible in the thigh [19].

Continuous Femoral nerve blockade can be established with the use of an indwelling perineural catheter. These are helpful for inpatients recovering from major hip surgery or amputations. There is evidence that continuous block in amputee patients can reduce the incidence of postoperative phantom limb sensation and pain [20]. One retrospective review of 198 patients that underwent a lower limb amputation for peripheral vascular disease found a 40% reduction in postoperative opioid use in patients that received a perineural catheter [21]. Commonly used solutions for continuous nerve blocks include 0.1–0.2% Ropivacaine or 0.25% Bupivacaine.

3.2.6 Saphenous Nerve Block

The saphenous nerve (SN) is the terminal sensory branch of the femoral nerve and carries dermatomes of L2–4 [22]. The saphenous nerve block is useful for surgeries involving the medial aspect of the lower leg and medial part of the ankle and foot as a supplement to general anesthesia. It can be blocked at various levels depends on surgical needs. The common sites used to block SN are peri-femoral below the inguinal crease, subsartorius at the femoral triangle and/or at the adductor canal, field block either at the medial femoral condyle or below the knee at the level of the tibial tuberosity, and at the medial side of the ankle as part of an ankle block [23]. The authors describe the three most common sites used for SN block.

3.2.6.1 Block Below the Knee

Local anesthetics administered using infiltration technique at the level of the tibial tuberosity, and this can be done by palpating the tibial tuberosity without the need for ultrasound. It is relatively easy to perform with less or no complications. Patient positioned with the leg straight. A subcutaneous wheel with 5–10 mL of local anesthetic injected the posterior aspect of the medial condyle of the tibia. Continuous catheter is not feasible at this site.

Indications Surgery at the medial aspect of the lower leg.

3.2.6.2 Adductor (Hunter's) Canal Block (ACB)

The adductor (Hunters's) canal is a space located deep to the sartorius muscle from the apex of the femoral triangle to the adductor hiatus [24]. The saphenous nerve passes through the adductor canal along with the femoral artery and vein. For the past more than a decade with increased utilization of US, this has become the most popular site to block SN. Moreover, the nerve to quadriceps muscles will be spared by choosing this method. Preservation of motor function around the knee is essential for most of the ambulatory procedures around the knee and lower leg. Van der Wal et al. first described the adductor canal block using surface landmarks [25], whereas Manickam et al. performed the adductor canal block for knee surgeries under ultrasound guidance [26].

Technique Ultrasound (US) is essential to locate various structures and to administer LA between mid and lower thigh. The patient is positioned supine, with the leg abducted at the hip and rotated externally, by using US mark the essential structures such as the femoral artery, vastus medialis muscle, and sartorius around SN (Fig. 3.14). Generally, the US probe placed between anterior superior iliac spine and

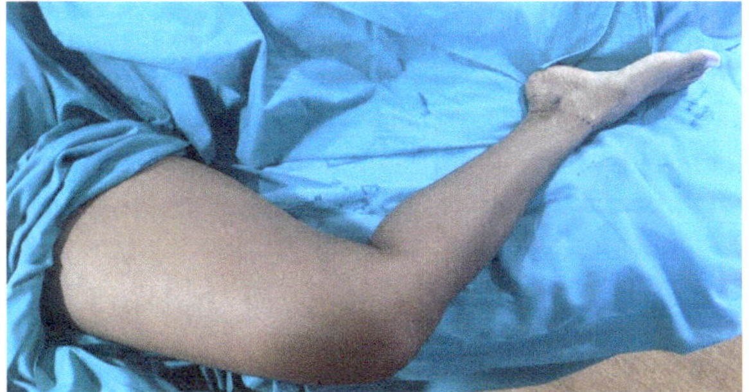

Frog leg positioning for Femoral nerve block and Adductor Canal block-abduction and external rotation at the hip, flexion at the knee

Fig. 3.14 Frog leg position for ACB

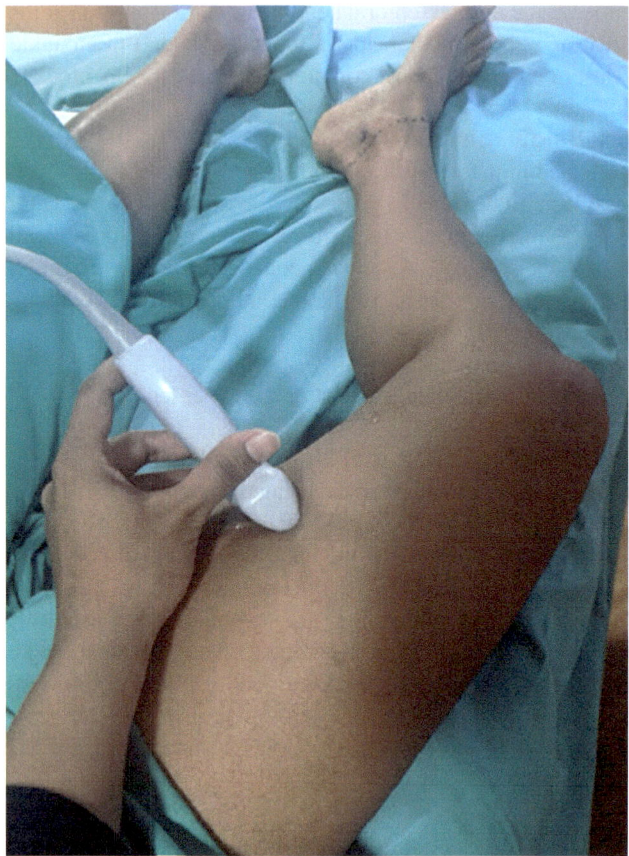

Fig. 3.15 Ultrasound position for ACB at mid thigh

patella (Fig. 3.15). SN lies close to the femoral artery at mid-thigh level (Fig. 3.16) and it separates from the superficial femoral artery as we move the US more distally, make it ideal to perform SN block. The needle can be entered either the medial or lateral aspect of the thigh, although it is advisable to do it from the lateral side at mid-thigh level to avoid inadvertent injury to femoral vessels (Fig. 3.17). Once desired location of SN identified, in-plane method is commonly used to track the needle, and after negative aspiration 10 mL of the desired local anesthetic is administered deeper to the sartorius muscle and lateral to the artery. In addition to the US, utilizing nerve stimulation will able to minimize block nerve to vastus medialis which lies just lateral to SN.

Indications Surgery at the knee, lower leg, and foot.

Potential complications Vascular injury can be prevented by appropriate location and negative aspiration. Muscle weakness especially with proximal thigh level

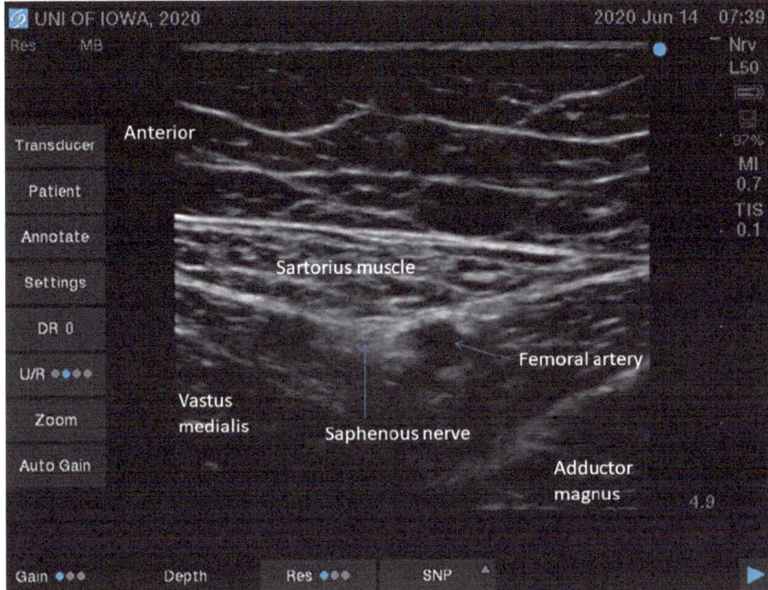

Ultrasonography of adductor canal block at mid-thigh

Fig. 3.16 Ultrasound showing relationship between femoral vessels and SN at the level of mid thigh

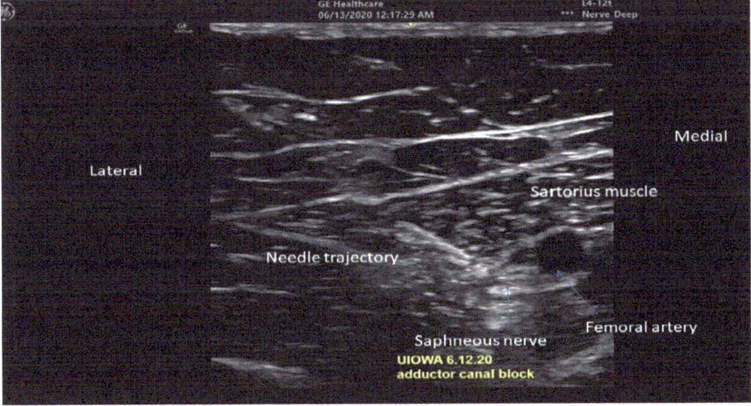

Fig. 3.17 Ultrasound image of ACB shows needle trajectory

blocking. Nerve injury, persistent paresthesia, or nerve entrapment usually occurs with distal thigh blocking.

Clinical Implications Studies have shown a wide range of success rates with ACB between 77 and 91% [27, 28]. The quality of block is affected by the site of the saphenous nerve block. Shain et al. in their comparative trail between medial infra-condylar and sub-sartorial approach showed a longer duration of blockade with sub-sartorial method. SN within the adductor canal allows a prolonged period of contact with LA [29]. Sztain et al. in their comparative trials between proximal and distal continuous ACB, showed less median and maximum pain score with the proximal insertion of catheter. However, there were no differences in ambulation and opioid consumption [30].

Several studies reported no incidences of quadriceps muscle weakness with ACB especially if you perform block at mid to distal thigh [31–33]. Jager et al. showed preserving quadriceps strength in 52% as compared to only 18% in the femoral nerve block group without affecting postoperative pain relief [16]. Zhang et al. in their meta-analysis from 11 studies (n-971) between FNB and ACB, observed similar outcomes with preservation of quadriceps muscle power without any significant differences in analgesic requirements or fall [34]. Similar observation from another meta-analysis (n-609) showed improved mobilization ability without compromising analgesia following knee arthroplasty [35]. Leung P et al. in their RCT from 70 patients observed superior pain control, less opioid consumption without significant difference in mobility in continuous ACB [36]. On the contrary, Kayupov et al. in their three-arm RCT showed less pain score ($p = 0.009$), early ambulation ($p = 0.02$), no differences in postoperative opioid consumption with continuous ACB compared to spinal, and combined spinal epidural analgesia groups for primary knee arthroplasty [37]. However, there have been reports of muscle weakness inevitable irrespective of the site of block [38]. Weismann et al. in their comparative study reported no superior effect of continuous ACB over FNB for early mobilization [39]. It is generally advisable to monitor motor weakness of the quadriceps to prevent movement-related injuries.

3.2.7 Sciatic Nerve Block

Sciatic nerve is the largest and thickest nerve in the body and it arises from the sciatic plexus and carries dermatomes of L4,5, S1,2, and 3 [40]. It provides sensory supply to the leg except for the thin medial strip which is innervated by the saphenous nerve. It can be blocked at multiple sites with different approaches. Victor Pauchet, a French surgeon, first described the sciatic nerve block in the 1920s. By combining with the posterior femoral cutaneous block, surgical anesthesia can be provided for the posterior aspect of the thigh and knee. Along with either femoral three in one or saphenous nerve block, analgesia can achieve for the anterior aspect of the thigh, knee, and lower leg. Onset time varies with LA between 10 (2% lidocaine) and 30 min (0.5% bupivacaine) and the duration of analgesia lasts up to 48 h.

Technique For high sciatic block posterior, various approaches such as classic posterior (Labat), gluteal, and para sacral modifications, lithotomy approach [41], or anterior approach [42] have been described [41–43]. Sciatic nerve block can be done with ultrasound-guided or nerve stimulation or a combination of both in certain approaches. In this chapter authors described commonly used approaches for sciatic nerve block.

Ultrasound-Guided Posterior Approach Patient needs to be positioned between lateral and prone with flexion of hip and knee. Sciatic nerve lies between the greater trochanter of the femur and ischial tuberosity. US transducer is held transverse to the course of the sciatic nerve. Two different methods are used for the posterior approach, either transgluteal or infragluteal. For transgluteal, the needle is inserted through the gluteus maximus and for infragluteal, the needle is placed just below the gluteal maximus.

Transgluteal Method First step is to identify the gluteus maximus, a superficial muscle lies between the ischial tuberosity and the greater trochanter of the femur. The sciatic nerve lies just deeper to the gluteus maximus. The Gluteus maximus lies superficial to the quadriceps femoris muscle and it is hyperechoic, flat and broad [44, 45].The needle is inserted in plane from the lateral aspect of the transducer and positioned with the tip of the needle adjacent to the nerve.

Infragluteal Approach For this approach first step is to identify the gluteus maximus and transducer is placed just below the level of the subgluteal crease. The sciatic nerve is located deep to the long head of the biceps femoris muscle and the posterior surface of the adductor magnus muscle at this location (Fig. 3.18). The needle is insertion is similar to transgluteal approach and in-plane method is commonly used to track the needle and positioned with the tip of the needle adjacent to the nerve [46].

For both approaches, the desired local anesthetic at 5 mL increment boluses with a total of 20 mL is injected after negative aspiration.

Nerve Stimulator-Guided Sciatic Block With growing interest of ultrasound technique, sciatic nerve block using nerve stimulation method rarely performed. It can be approached in either the prone or lateral decubitus positions. If the Labat, classic lateral decubitus position is used, anatomic landmarks including the PSIS, greater trochanter, and sacral hiatus are identified and marked (Fig. 3.19). An oblique line is drawn between the PSIS and the greater trochanter. A second line is drawn from the greater trochanter to the sacral hiatus. The third line about 3–5 cm drawn between the first and second line and it is bisected between these two lines. The insulated needle is inserted at the intersection of these last two lines (lines 2 and 3), perpendicular to the skin, until plantar flexion is achieved at 0.5 mA [3]. Approximately 20 mL of LA is injected in 5 mL increments after negative aspiration, with gentle aspiration between injections. If the prone position is used, the needle is inserted just lateral to the ischial tuberosity and advanced until plantar flexion is achieved at 0.5 mA.

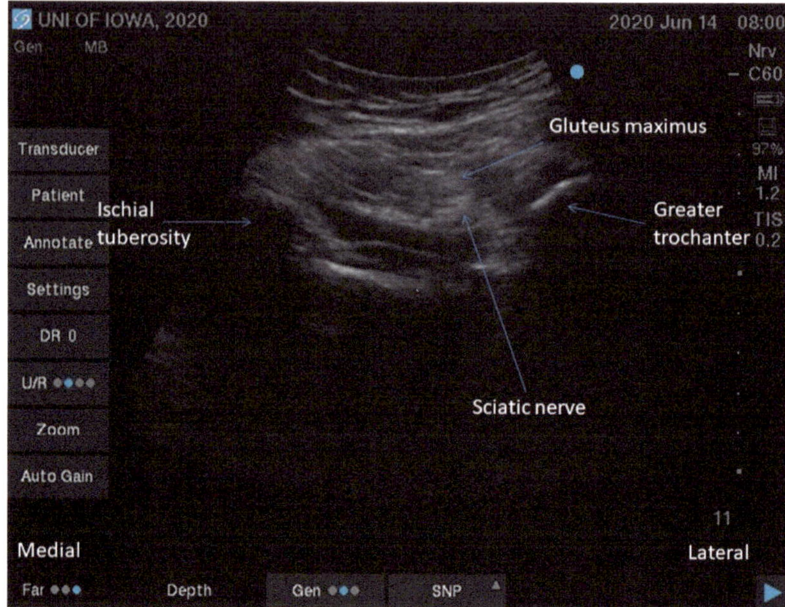

Fig. 3.18 Ultrasound image of the sciatic nerve at the infragluteal region

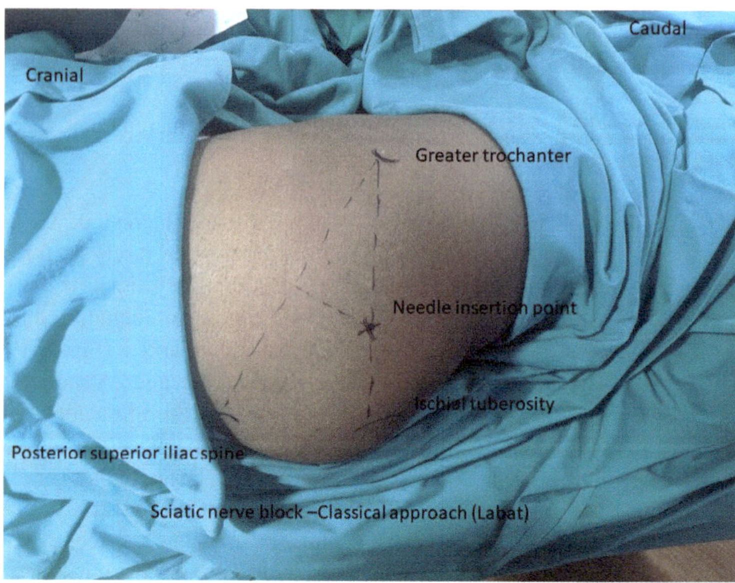

Fig. 3.19 Patient positioning and anatomic landmarks for lateral approach for sciatic nerve block

Anterior Approach This method is rarely used in current clinical practice. However, it is very useful in patients with significant motion restriction at hip and knees, especially, secondary to acute injury. This method is commonly performed by using both ultrasound and nerve stimulation. A curvilinear (2–8 MHz) ultrasound probe is placed over the anteromedial thigh, 2–3 cm caudad to the inguinal ligament. The first step is to identify the femoral artery and profunda femoris artery which is a deeper structure. The sciatic nerve is visualized as a hyperechoic, flattened oval structure between the adductor magnus and hamstring muscles, medial to the femur, a usually at a depth of 6–8 cm (Fig. 3.20). Typically, a 100 mm, 21 or 22 gage insulated needle is inserted in-plane in a medial-to-lateral direction and advanced toward the sciatic nerve. The calf or foot muscle motor response should be obtained at 0.5 mA with the nerve stimulator. After successful negative aspiration, 1–2 mL of LA is injected, visualizing spread around the sciatic nerve. The needle reposition is required if there is insufficient spread of the LA around the nerve. Total of 15–20 mL of LA is injected in 5-mL increments, with gentle aspiration between injections [47].

Perineural Catheter Sciatic Block Continuous sciatic nerve block for extended pain relief for certain surgeries involves knee, ankle, or foot. The technique for placing the indwelling perineural catheter is the same as for single-shot injections, using ultrasound guidance or nerve stimulation [48–50].

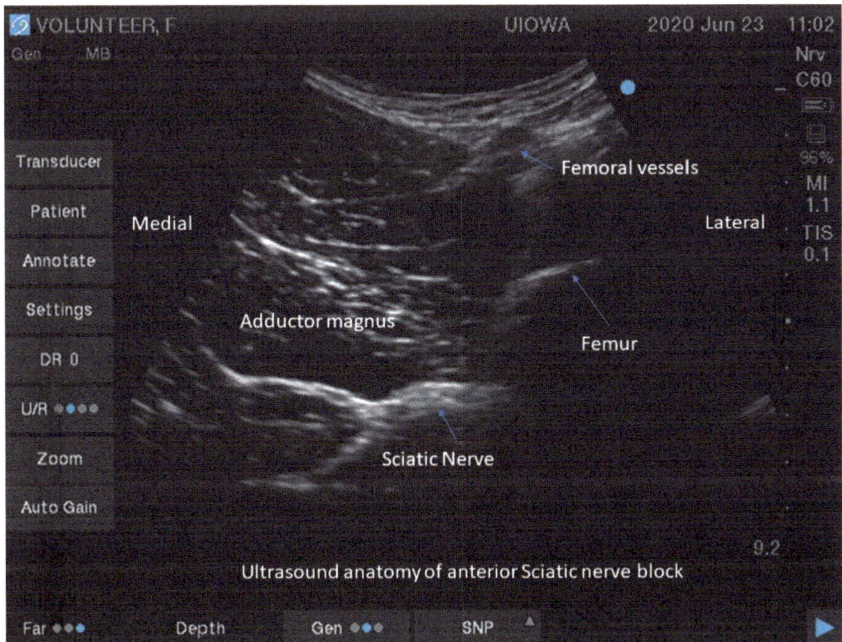

Fig. 3.20 Ultrasound image showing an anterior approach for sciatic nerve block

Indications High sciatic nerve block irrespective of approach, provides analgesia for surgery on the thigh (along with femoral or saphenous nerve block), knee, foot, or ankle (along with saphenous nerve block).

Potential Complications Inadvertent vascular injuries, infection especially with a continuous nerve block, nerve injury, and persistent paresthesia due to close proximity to bony prominences such as ischial tuberosity and greater trochanter of femur.

3.2.7.1 Clinical Implications

Comparing Various Approaches

Several studies reported differences in the onset, quality of blockade, and patient satisfaction between various approaches. Taboada et al. in their comparative study between classic posterior modified subgluteal, and lateral popliteal approaches showed early onset of sensory and motor blockade with 0.75% ropivacaine in the first two approaches [51]. Posterior approach has a shorter onset time (7.5 vs. 12.5 min), better patient satisfaction and analgesic quality compared to the anterior approach [52]. Tammam et al. in their comparative study of four different approaches (short and long axis in-plane and short and long axis out-of-plane ultrasound technique) in the infragluteal region demonstrated rapid onset of the blockade and better patient satisfaction with the long axis in-plane method [53].

Comparing Ultrasound Guided Versus Nerve Stimulation Methods

Compared to nerve stimulation method, ultrasound-guided sciatic nerve block, provided higher success rate [RR = 1.22 95% CI: 1.04–1.42, $p = 0.01$] from the meta-nalysis (n = 10 studies). In addition, USG reduces the risk of vascular puncture [RR = 0.13 95% CI: 0.02–0.97, $p = 0.05$], however no significant difference observed in the success rate of catheter placement [RR = 1.1095% CI: 0.93–1.29, $p = 0.27$] or the time of performing sciatica never block [RR = −0.17 95% CI: −1.61–1.27, $p = 0.82$] [54]. In another comparative study, demonstrated 37% reduction in the minimum effective volume (MEAV50) of 1.5% mepivacaine (12 vs. 19 mL) required to block the sciatic nerve compared to nerve stimulation method without significant difference in the quality of blockade [55]. Overall USG block has potential benefits.

Combined Femoral and Sciatic Nerve Block

Utilizing combined femoral and sciatic nerve block for patients with significant comorbidities, potentially high risk for general anesthesia, has been reported as a sole anesthetic with minimal sedation [56]. This combined technique has been used for various knee procedures. A metanalysis from seven studies ($n = 617$) showed an earlier onset of blockade when sciatic NB combined with femoral NB as compared to femoral NB and local infiltration around the knee. However, there were no meaningful differences in terms of active knee flexion, length of hospital stay, morphine use, PONV, and the occurrence of fall between groups [57]. In the pediatric population, for ACL reconstruction, combined block showed superior pain control, reduce opioid requirements in the immediate postoperative period, and shorter length of stay in the PACU compared to femoral NB alone.

Posterior Femoral Cutaneous Nerve Block
The posterior femoral cutaneous nerve (PFCN) is one of six branches directly arises from the sacral plexus, prior to its convergence into anterior and posterior divisions. It arises from the posterior divisions of the anterior rami of S1 and S2 nerves and the anterior divisions of anterior rami of S2 and S3 nerves. PFCN runs along the sciatic nerve below the gluteus maximus and above the biceps femoris. To identify PFCN approaches used for sciatic nerve can be implemented, and often time with a large volume of local anesthetic, PFCN received sufficient LA during high sciatic nerve block [58, 59]. However, in certain circumstances such as surgery involves upper posterior aspect of the thigh, and or any procedures at the knee, ankle, or foot warranting tourniquet at upper thigh, it is essential to selectively block the PFCN. Although analgesic requirements for tourniquet pain are controversial, a prospective study on the continuous sciatic block at popliteal level without PFCN observed no significant requirements of opioids [60].

3.2.8 Popliteal Sciatic Nerve Block

Popliteal approach is used to block the sciatic nerve just prior to its terminal branches tibial and common fibular (peroneal) nerves. For this method, either ultrasound-guided or nerve stimulation or combinations of both are used. Some studies showed an early onset of the blockade with the ultrasound method [61, 62]. Three commonly used approaches are lateral, prone, or supine based on patient's mobility restriction.

Ultrasound-Guided Block For this method, the patient generally positioned lateral decubitus with slight flexion at the leg. If block can be performed only in supine, the calf and foot need to be elevated using stand or pillows, the hip is flexed at approximately 45 degrees and the knee is flexed 90 degrees for access to the popliteal fossa and distal posterior thigh. Probe can also be placed anteriorly to visualize the popliteal with challenges in certain patient population. For the prone position, pillow can be placed under the ankle to flex the knee for better access. Irrespective of patient position, the first step is to identify popliteal crease and popliteal fossa, and by having the patient flex the knee helps visualize the popliteal crease. Then the ultrasound probe is placed over the popliteal crease in an axial orientation and the popliteal artery is visualized as an initial landmark (Fig. 3.21). The tibial nerve lies superficial to the popliteal artery and the popliteal vein lies between the popliteal artery and the tibial nerve, easily compressible but often difficult to visualize. The ultrasound transducer moved proximally by following the tibial nerve until to the branch point of the sciatic nerve; where the common fibular nerve is visualized, lateral to the tibial nerve (Fig. 3.22). The sciatic nerve bifurcates approximately 6–7 cm above the popliteal crease in adults, but it varies widely. The block generally performed proximal or distal to this bifurcation. The sciatic nerve is hyperechoic and visualized between the biceps femoris and semitendinosus/semimembranosus

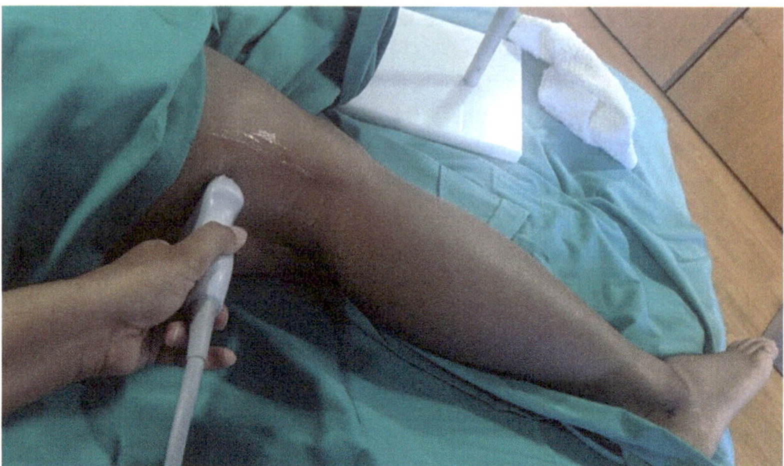

Probe position for Ultraasound guided sciatic block in popliteal fossa

Fig. 3.21 Ultrasound probe position for popliteal sciatic nerve block

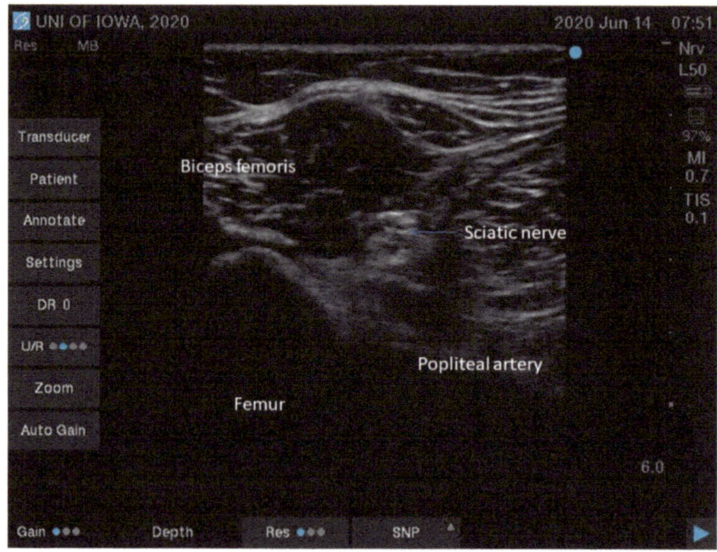

Ultrasonography of sciatic nerve in the popliteal fossa

Fig. 3.22 Ultrasound image shows sciatic nerve at the popliteal fossa

tendons. In-plane technique is commonly used for this method and an 80–100 mm needle is inserted in the lateral thigh parallel to the transducer and directed toward the hyperechoic nerve. 20–30 mL of local anesthetic (LA) is injected in 5 mL increments after negative aspiration, with gentle aspiration between injections.

In general, the circumferential spread of LA should be visualized around the entire sciatic nerve or around each of the two branches. Studies have shown the early onset of the blockade with circumferential spread, as well as injection distal to the sciatic bifurcation, as compared to blocking sciatic nerve proximally [63, 64]. Para neural sheath around the sciatic nerve can be visualized easily with ultrasound and having this sheath facilitates the spread of local anesthetics [65].

Nerve Stimulator-Guided Popliteal Block For this method, either a lateral or a posterior needle approach is implemented. For the lateral approach, the patient needs to be positioned supine with the calf supported on a stand, similar to US method. The needle is inserted in the lateral thigh, between the biceps femoris and the vastus lateralis muscles. The needle then directed toward the femur, once in contact with the femur needle needs to be withdrawn to the skin, reoriented at a 30 degree angle from the horizontal aiming posteriorly, and advanced while looking for nerve response. For the posterior approach patient is positioned prone. The first step is to identify semitendinosus/semimembranosus muscles in the medial aspect and biceps femoris in the lateral aspect of the thigh. The insulated needle is inserted at the center point between these tendons, approximately 6–7 cm above the popliteal crease. After eliciting either plantar flexion or inversion of the foot, the stimulating intensity is reduced until twitch is maintained at 0.4 mA [66]. If no response is initially achieved, the needle is moved laterally. After negative aspiration, 30 mL of LA is injected in 5 mL increments, with gentle aspiration between injections.

3.2.8.1 Clinical Implications

One of the challenges with popliteal sciatic nerve block is to localize the desired site for injection. Several studies reported varying anatomy of sciatic nerve bifurcation into tibial and common peroneal nerves. Determining the course of the sciatic nerve with appropriate ultrasound imaging is essential for successful block [67]. Multiple studies have demonstrated that, for single-injection popliteal sciatic nerve blocks, block characteristics are dependent upon local anesthetic injection relative to the sciatic nerve bifurcation. A dual center RCT, observed superior pain control for continuous NB if the tip of the catheter placed 5 cm proximal to the bifurcation sciatic nerve and if the site of injection distal to bifurcation in single-injection group. However, no differences in terms of opioid consumption, neuropathic symptoms or infection-related complications between groups [68].

Comparison Between USG and Nerve Stimulation Methods

Many studies demonstrated significant benefits with USG popliteal sciatic NB compared to the nerve stimulation technique. In obese patients, USG lateral popliteal nerve block was superior in terms of shorter procedure time (206 vs. 577 s, $p < 0.001$), les number of needle repositions, and less procedure-related pain [69]. In a prospective RCT, USG popliteal SNB reduces the required dose of local anesthetic significantly and is also associated with a higher success rate compared to nerve stimulation without significantly affecting block characteristics [70]. In a metanalysis from five RCT, continuous SNB in comparison with single shot, showed better pain control at 24 and 48 h after ambulatory foot and ankle surgery. There was no difference in neuropathic or infection-related complications between groups, however, drug leakage was experienced in 13.9% in continuous NB group [71].

3.2.9 Infiltration of Local Anesthetic Between Popliteal Artery and Capsule of the Knee Block (IPACK)

The IPACK block is one of the relatively new blocks, thanks to the advancement of ultrasound technique. Ultrasound is essential to perform this block. The primary intention is to block sensory articular branches of the sciatic, tibial, common fibular, and posterior division of the obturator nerve. IPACK preserves motor function around knee and leg. As the name implies, it is a type of field block. Local anesthetics injected between the posterior aspect of the femur and popliteal artery.

Technique A low-frequency curvilinear ultrasound transducer is essential for this block. This block can be performed with the patient in either supine or prone position with slight flexion at the knee and leg needs to be supported. The first step is to locate the popliteal crease. The ultrasound transducer placed transverse orientation either posteriorly or postero-medially in the popliteal crease (Fig. 3.23). Then to identify the popliteal artery with 2D or using color doppler and the distal part of the femur. Transducer needs to be moved proximally if femoral condyles are visualized until the distal part of the shaft of femur visualized and it appears as flat surface. Sometimes at this level, tibial and common peroneal nerves may be identified. In-plane technique is recommended for needle insertion. An 80–100 mm needle is inserted from medial to lateral, in the space between the popliteal artery and the shaft of the femur. The needle insertion is typically parallel to the femur. The needle needs to be advanced until the tip is approximately 2 cm beyond the popliteal artery.

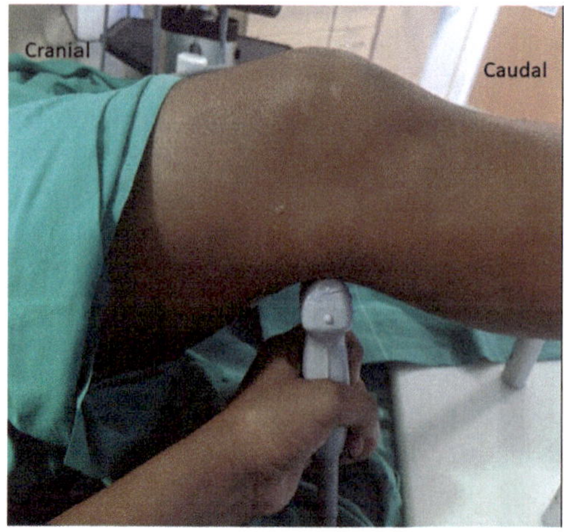

Fig. 3.23 Patient and ultrasound positioning for IPACK

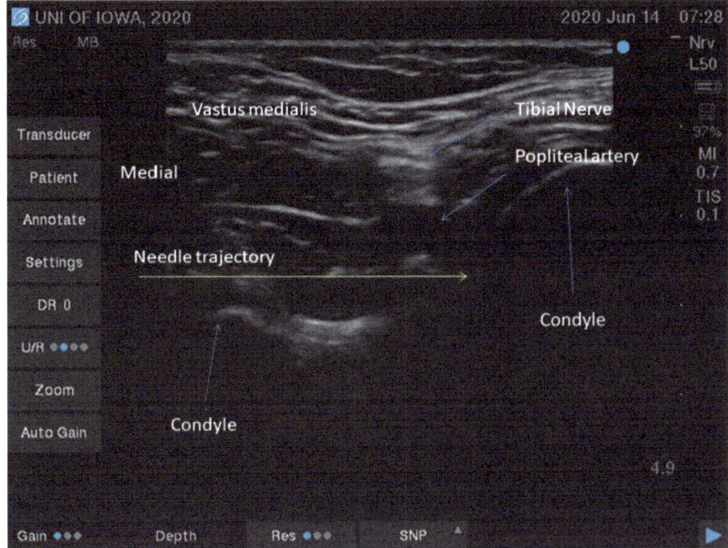

Fig. 3.24 Ultrasound image and needle trajectory for IPACK

One–two mL of LA injected as a test dose to ensure the development of hydro-dissection and to confirm the tip of the needle at the most desired location, space between the femur and popliteal artery (Fig. 3.24). After the negative aspiration and achievement of proper hydro-dissection, a total of 20 mL of LA is then infiltrated in the tissue plane. Being a limited space, it is recommended to gradually withdrawn the needle after each increment bolus of 5 mL. This technique facilitates uniform distribution of LA evenly between the initial needle tip location (2 cm lateral to the popliteal artery) and the posteromedial border of the femur.

Indications The IPACK block is used as supplemental analgesia following total knee arthroplasty, anterior cruciate ligament repair, and procedures that involve the posterior capsule of the knee with preservation of motor function around the knee [72, 73]. There are several ongoing trials to compare the efficacy of IPACK, adductor canal block, and infiltration around the knee by surgeons.

3.2.10 Ankle Block

Ankle block is a purely sensory block and it is achieved by block five nerves separately. Out of five nerves, four arises from the sciatic nerve, tibial, superficial, and deep peroneal [fibular] nerves, and sural nerve from medial to lateral, and one cutaneous branch from the femoral nerve (saphenous nerve).

Technique Ankle block can be performed with landmark based, anatomic technique, although ultrasound may be useful to locate deep peroneal, tibial, and sural nerves. Moreover, studies shown a higher success rate of ankle block with ultrasound in non-diabetic patients. In some circumstances instead of blocking all five nerves, desired nerves can be blocked as per surgical needs. There is no specific order of blocking the nerves although recommended first to block deeper nerves (tibial, deep peroneal and sural) and then superficial nerves such as superficial peroneal and saphenous nerves. Supine position with elevation of the foot and supported on blankets or pillows are preferred. The ankle needs to be rotated as needed to block all five nerves.

Tibial Nerve Block The distal part of the tibial nerve provides sensory supply to calcaneus and medal part of the plantar surface of the sole. Tibial nerve can be blocked either by the landmark method or using ultrasound.

Landmark Anatomical Method First step to palpate the posterior tibial artery which lies between the medial malleolus of tibia and the tip of calcaneus. The 2 in. hypodermic needle inserted just posterior to the posterior tibial artery at 45 degrees aiming toward the medial malleolus (Fig. 3.25). Once needle is in contact with the bone, 2–3 mL LA injected after slight withdrawal. The needle then repositions both medially and laterally to inject another 2 mL, to create fan-shaped infiltration to improve the success rate of the block.

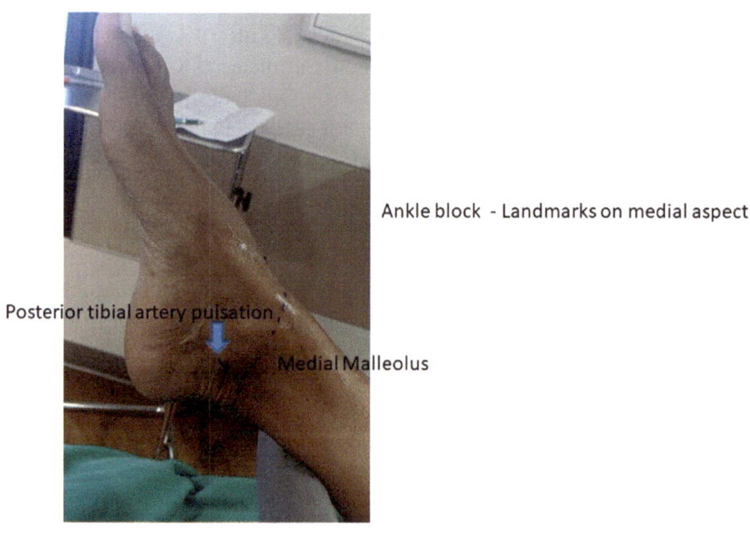

Fig. 3.25 Anatomic landmark and needle insertion site for tibial nerve block

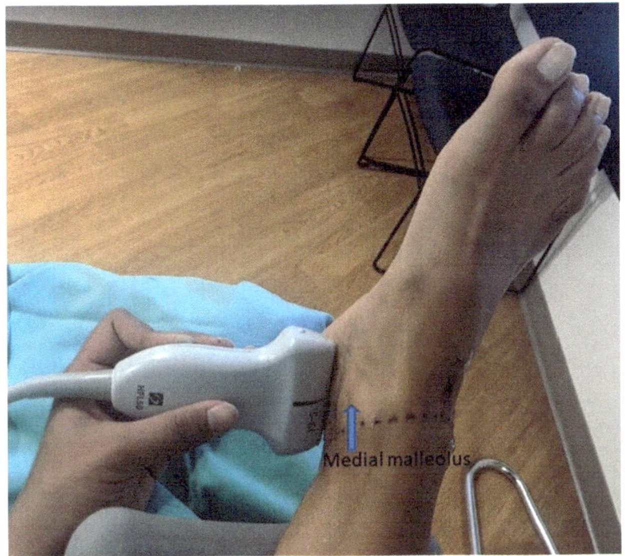

Ultrasound probe position for Tibial Nerve block

Fig. 3.26 Ultrasound probe position for tibial nerve block

Ultrasound-Guided Method The ultrasound probe was placed in the transverse orientation just above the medial malleolus to visualize the posterior tibial artery with 2D or color doppler (Fig. 3.26). The tibial nerve located posterior to the posterior tibial artery and the needle is inserted similar to the landmark technique aiming toward the nerve and it can either in-plane or out of the plane (Fig. 3.27). A 3–5 mL of LA injected around the nerve to create a circumferential spread for successful blockade [74].

Indications Surgery involves medial aspect of the ankle and foot.

3.2.11 Saphenous Nerve Block

Saphenous nerve gives sensory supply to the medial part of the ankle and foot. It is a superficial nerve that lies close to the saphenous vein and easy to block with subcutaneous infiltration around the medial malleolus by injecting 3–5 mL of local anesthetics. The needle preferable directed toward Achilles tendon for the complete blockade. Ultrasound rarely required for this block. Saphenous vein used as reference structure to perform saphenous nerve block with this technique. 2–3 mL is sufficient for US-guided block.

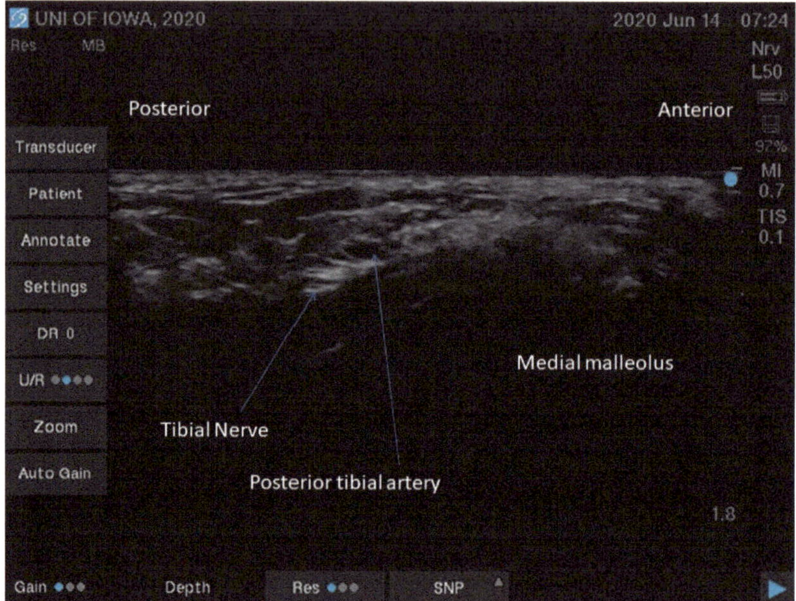

Ultrasonography of Tibial Nerve block at ankle

Fig. 3.27 Ultrasound image of the tibial nerve at the ankle

Indications Surgery involves the medial aspect of the foot and ankle. Along with popliteal sciatic nerve block, this block can provide complete analgesia for all foot and ankle surgeries.

3.2.12 Superficial Peroneal Nerve Block

Superficial peroneal nerve innervates the whole dorsum of foot except for the first web space. It is a superficial nerve, blocked by subcutaneous infiltration of 5 mL of local anesthetics by inserting needle between two malleoli and directed toward each malleolus.

Indications Surgery involves forefoot and toes.

3.2.13 Deep Peroneal Nerve Block

Deep peroneal nerve supplies the dorsum of the foot at the first web space. The block is performed with either landmark anatomical method or using ultrasound.

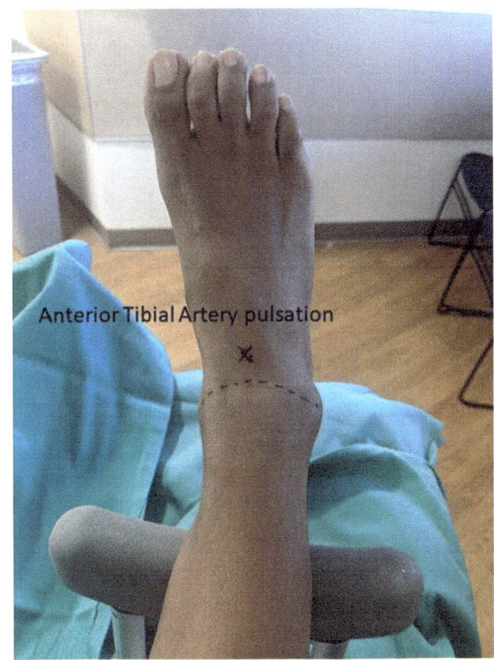

Fig. 3.28 Anatomic landmark for deep peroneal nerve

Landmark Method The first step is to palpate the dorsalis pedis artery which lies between extensor hallucis longus and extensor digitorum longus tendons. These two tendons get prominent with dorsiflexion of the great toe. The deep peroneal nerve lies just lateral to the dorsalis pedis artery (Fig. 3.28). This block is performed at the midtarsal level by inserting hypodermic needle lateral to the artery until it contacts the tarsal bone. A 2–3 mL of LA is injected after slight withdrawal of the needle from bony contact.

Ultrasound Method Patient position is similar to the landmark technique. Place the ultrasound transducer in transverse orientation at the mid dorsum level (Fig. 3.29). Visualize the dorsalis pedis artery with 2D or color doppler (Fig. 3.30). A hypodermic needle was inserted lateral to the artery in in-plane orientation and blockade achieved with 2–3 mL of LA. Occasionally, the extensor hallucis longus tendon misidentified as nerve, and by dorsi of the great toe will able to differentiate between tendon and nerve.

Indications Surgery involves the medial aspect of the forefoot, and first and second toe.

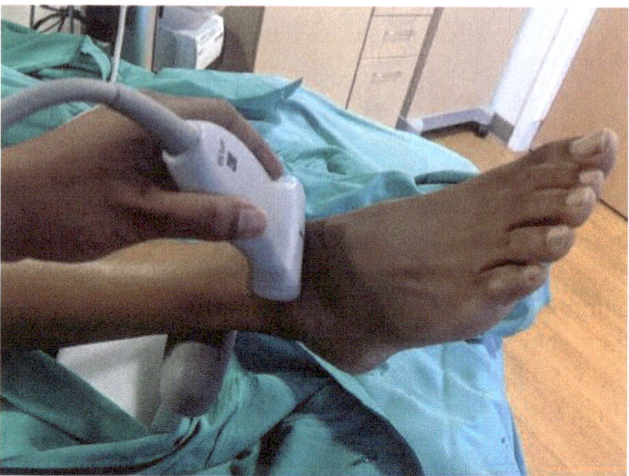

Fig. 3.29 Ultrasound position for deep peroneal nerve

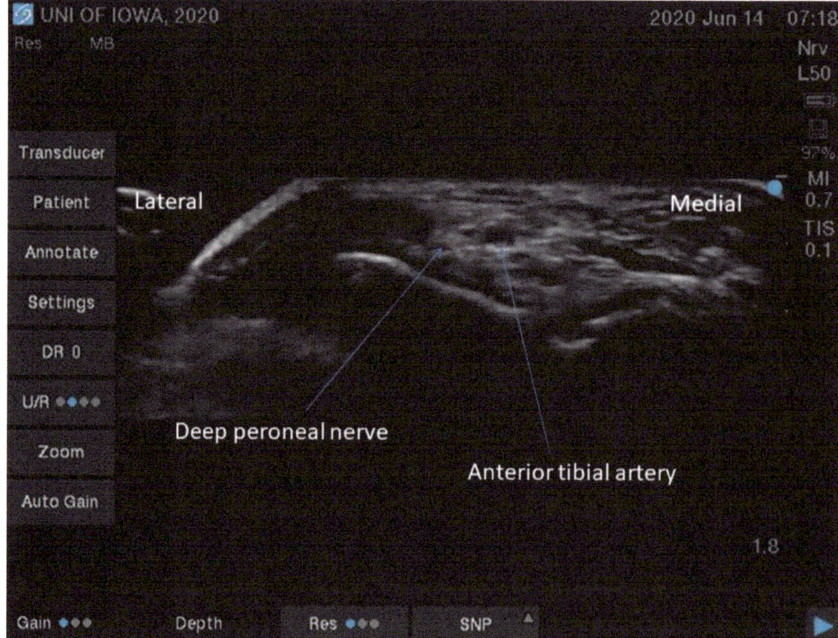

Fig. 3.30 Ultrasound image shows deep peroneal nerve block

3.2.14 Sural Nerve Block

The sural nerve innervates the lateral aspect of the ankle, foot, and fifth toe. It typically runs posterior to lateral malleolus in the subcutaneous plane. Sural nerve block is achieved with landmark anatomical method or using ultrasound. For the anatomical method, hypodermic needle inserted posterior to lateral malleolus until it

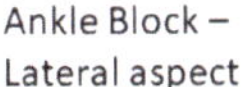

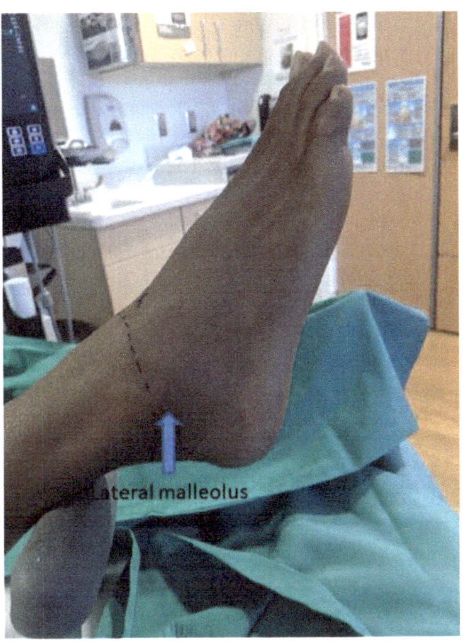

Fig. 3.31 Anatomic landmark technique of sural nerve block

contacts with bone, 5 mL of LA injected in wheel fashion after slight withdrawal from the bone (Fig. 3.31). Ultrasound transducer is positioned in the transverse plane just above the lateral malleolus to visualize the hyperechoic sural nerve. Lesser saphenous vein used as a reference structure in challenging circumstances and the nerve lies next to the vein [75]. Blockade was achieved with 5 mL of LA around the nerve after confirmation of negative aspiration.

Indications Surgery involves the lateral aspect of the ankle, foot, and fifth toe.

3.2.14.1 Clinical Implications

Ankle block has been widely used for forefoot and various surgeries in the toes especially in high-risk patients for general anesthesia with the presence of significant comorbidities. However, it has its own challenges/limitations with significant edematous tissue around the ankle. Posterior tibial nerve block has been performed predominantly in the para-malleolar area without USG/nerve stimulation with early onset compared to the proximal part of the tibial nerve block (8 vs. 13 min). However, in patients with restricted access, the proximal approach may be a useful alternative technique [76].

References

1. Borghi B, D'Addabbo M, White PF, Gallerani P, Toccaceli L, Raffaeli W, et al. The use of prolonged peripheral neural blockade after lower extremity amputation: the effect on symptoms associated with phantom limb syndrome. Anesth Analg. 2010;111(5):1308–15.

2. Brull R, McCartney CJ, Chan VW, El-Beheiry H. Neurological complications after regional anesthesia: contemporary estimates of risk. Anesth Analg. 2007;104(4):965–74.
3. Koh M, Markovich B. Anatomy, abdomen and pelvis, obturator nerve. [Updated 2019 Dec 11]. In: StatPearls [Internet]. Treasure Island, FL: StatPearls Publishing; 2020. https://www.ncbi.nlm.nih.gov/books/NBK551640/.
4. Giuffre BA, Jeanmonod R. Anatomy, sciatic nerve. [Updated 2020 Apr 23]. In: StatPearls [Internet]. Treasure Island, FL: StatPearls Publishing; 2020. https://www.ncbi.nlm.nih.gov/books/NBK482431/.
5. Sabnis AS. Anatomical variations of sciatic nerve bifurcation in human cadavers. J Clin Res Lett. 2012;3(2):46–8.
6. Walji AH, Tsui BCH. Clinical anatomy of the sacral plexus. In: Tsui B, Suresh S, editors. Pediatric atlas of ultrasound- and nerve stimulation-guided regional anesthesia. New York, NY: Springer; 2016.
7. Touray ST, de Leeuw MA, Zuurmond WW, Perez RS. Psoas compartment block for lower extremity surgery: a meta-analysis. Br J Anaesth. 2008;101:750–60.
8. Morimoto M, Kim JT, Popovic J, Jain S, Bekker A. Ultrasound-guided lumbar plexus block for open reduction and internal fixation of hip fracture. Pain Pract. 2006;6(2):124–6.
9. Klein SM, D'Ercole F, Greengrass RA, Warner DS. Enoxaparin associated with psoas hematoma and lumbar plexopathy after lumbar plexus block. Anesthesiology. 1997;87:1576–9.
10. Weller RS, Gerancher JC, Crews JC, Wade KL. Extensive retroperitoneal hematoma without neurologic deficit in two patients who underwent lumbar plexus block and were later anticoagulated. Anesthesiology. 2003;98(2):581–5.
11. de Visme V, Picart F, Le Jouan R, Legrand A, Savry C, Morin V. Combined lumbar and sacral plexus block compared with plain bupivacaine spinal anesthesia for hip fractures in the elderly. Reg Anesth Pain Med. 2000;25:158–62.
12. Ilfeld BM, Ball ST, Gearen PF, Le LT, Mariano ER, Vandenborne K, et al. Ambulatory continuous posterior lumbar plexus nerve blocks after hip arthroplasty: a dual-center, randomized, triple-masked, placebo-controlled trial. Anesthesiology. 2008;109(3):491–501.
13. Amiri HR, Safari S, Makarem J, Rahimi M, Jahanshahi B. Comparison of combined femoral nerve block and spinal anesthesia with lumbar plexus block for postoperative analgesia in intertrochanteric fracture surgery. Anesth Pain Med. 2012;2(1):32–5.
14. Nie H, Yang YX, Wang Y, Liu Y, Zhao B, Luan B. Effects of continuous fascia iliaca compartment blocks for postoperative analgesia in patients with hip fracture. Pain Res Manag. 2015;20(4):210–2.
15. Newman B, McCarthy L, Thomas PW, May P, Layzell M, Horn K. A comparison of preoperative nerve stimulator-guided femoral nerve block and fascia iliaca compartment block in patients with a femoral neck fracture. Anaesthesia. 2013;68(9):899–903.
16. Jæger P, Zaric D, Fomsgaard JS, Hilsted KL, Bjerregaard J, Gyrn J, et al. Adductor canal block versus femoral nerve block for analgesia after total knee arthroplasty: a randomized, double-blind study. Reg Anesth Pain Med. 2013;38(6):526–32.
17. Szűcs S, Morau D, Sultan SF, Iohom G, Shorten G. A comparison of three techniques (local anesthetic deposited circumferential to vs. above vs. below the nerve) for ultrasound guided femoral nerve block. BMC Anesthesiol. 2014;14:6.
18. Turbitt LR, McHardy PG, Casanova M, Shapiro J, Li L, Choi S. Analysis of inpatient falls after total knee arthroplasty in patients with continuous femoral nerve block. Anesth Analg. 2018;127(1):224–7.
19. Grevstad U, Mathiesen O, Valentiner LS, Jaeger P, Hilsted KL, Dahl JB. Effect of adductor canal block versus femoral nerve block on quadriceps strength, mobilization, and pain after total knee arthroplasty: a randomized, blinded study. Reg Anesth Pain Med. 2015;40:3–10.
20. Morey TE, Giannoni J, Duncan E, Scarborough MT, Enneking FK. Nerve sheath catheter analgesia after amputation. Clin Orthop Relat Res. 2002;397:281–9.
21. Aylinga OG, Montbriandb J, Jiang S, Ladak S, Love L, Eisenberg N, et al. Continuous regional anaesthesia provides effective pain management and reduces opioid requirement following major lower limb amputation. Eur J Vasc Endovasc Surg. 2014;48(5):559–64.

22. Williams PL, Bannister LH. Gray's anatomy: the anatomical basis of medicine and surgery. 38th ed. New York: Churchill Livingstone; 1995.
23. Benzon HT, Sharma S, Calimaran A. Comparison of the different approaches to saphenous nerve block. Anesthesiology. 2005;102:633–8.
24. Roamnes GJ, editor. Cunningham's Textbook of anatomy. 12th ed. New York: Oxford Medical Publications; 1981.
25. van der Wal M, Lang SA, Yip RW. Transsartorial approach for saphenous nerve block. Can J Anaesth. 1993;40:542–6.
26. Manickam B, Perlas A, Duggan E, Brull R, Chan VW, Ramlogan R. Feasibility and efficacy of ultrasound-guided block of the saphenous nerve in the adductor canal. Reg Anesth Pain Med. 2009;34:578–80.
27. Head SJ, Leung RC, Hackman GP, Seib R, Rondi K, Schwarz SK. Ultrasound-guided saphenous nerve block – Within versus distal to the adductor canal: a proof-of-principle randomized trial. Can J Anaesth. 2015;62:37–44.
28. Tsai PB, Karnwal A, Kakazu C, Tokhner V, Julka IS. Efficacy of an ultrasound-guided subsartorial approach to saphenous nerve block: a case series. Can J Anaesth. 2010;57:683–8.
29. Sahin L, Eken ML, Isik M, Cavus O. Comparison of infracondylar versus subsartorial approach to saphenous nerve block: a randomized controlled study. Anaesthesiology. 2017;11(3):287–92.
30. Sztain JF, Khatibi B, Monahan AM, Said ET, Abramson WB, Gabriel RA, et al. Proximal versus distal continuous adductor canal blocks: does varying perineural catheter location influence analgesia? A randomized, subject-masked, controlled clinical trial. Anesth Analg. 2018;127(1):240–6.
31. Kwofie MK, Shastri UD, Gadsden JC, Sinha SK, Abrams JH, Xu D, et al. The effects of ultrasound-guided adductor canal block versus femoral nerve block on quadriceps strength and fall risk: a blinded, randomized trial of volunteers. Reg Anesth Pain Med. 2013;38:321–5.
32. Davis JJ, Bond TS, Swenson JD. Adductor canal block: more than just the saphenous nerve? Reg Anesth Pain Med. 2009;34:618–9.
33. Abdallah FW, Whelan DB, Chan VW, Prasad GA, Endersby RV, Theodoropolous J, et al. Adductor canal block provides noninferior analgesia and superior quadriceps strength compared with femoral nerve block in anterior cruciate ligament reconstruction. Anesthesiology. 2016;124:1053–64.
34. Zhang Z, Wang Y, Liu Y. Effectiveness of continuous adductor canal block versus continuous femoral nerve block in patients with total knee arthroplasty: a PRISMA guided systematic review and meta-analysis. Medicine (Baltimore). 2019;98(48):e18056.
35. Kuang MJ, Ma JX, Fu L, He WW, Zhao J, Ma XL. Is adductor canal block better than femoral nerve block in primary total knee arthroplasty? A GRADE analysis of the evidence through a systematic review and meta-analysis. J Arthroplasty. 2017;32(10):3238–48.
36. Leung P, Dickerson DM, Denduluri SK, Mohammed MK, Lu M, Anitescu M, Luu HH. Postoperative continuous adductor canal block for total knee arthroplasty improves pain and functional recovery: a randomized controlled clinical trial. J Clin Anesth. 2018;49:46–52.
37. Kayupov E, Okroj K, Young AC, Moric M, Luchetti TJ, Zisman G, et al. Continuous adductor canal blocks provide superior ambulation and pain control compared to epidural analgesia for primary knee arthroplasty: a randomized, controlled trial. J Arthroplasty. 2018;33(4):1040–4.
38. Chen J, Lesser JB, Hadzic A, Reiss W, Resta-Flarer F. Adductor canal block can result in motor block of the quadriceps muscle. Reg Anesth Pain Med. 2014;39:170–1.
39. Wiesmann T, Piechowiak K, Duderstadt S, Haupt D, Schmitt J, Eschbach D, et al. Continuous adductor canal block versus continuous femoral nerve block after total knee arthroplasty for mobilisation capability and pain treatment: a randomised and blinded clinical trial. Arch Orthop Trauma Surg. 2016;136(3):397–406.
40. Moore KL, Dalley AF, Agur AMR. Clinically oriented anatomy. 7th ed. Lippincott Williams & Wilkins: Baltimore, MD; 2014.
41. Labat G. Regional anesthesia: its technique and clinical applications. 2nd ed. Philadelphia, PA: WB Saunders; 1928. p. 45.

42. Beck GP. Anterior approach to sciatic nerve block. Anesthesiology. 1963;24:222–4.
43. Raj PP, Parks RI, Watson TD, Jenkins MT. A new single-position supine approach to sciatic-femoral nerve block. Anesth Analg. 1975;54:489–93.
44. Chan VW, Nova H, Abbas S, McCartney CJL, Perlas A, Xu DQ. Ultrasound examination and localization of the sciatic nerve: a volunteer study. Anesthesiology. 2006;104:309–14.
45. Graif M, Seton A, Nerubai J, Horoszowski H, Itzchak Y. Sciatic nerve: sonographic evaluation and anatomic-pathologic considerations. Radiology. 1991;181:405–8.
46. di Benedetto P, Casati A, Bertini L, Fanelli G. Posterior subgluteal approach to block the sciatic nerve: description of the technique and initial clinical experiences. Eur J Anaesthesiol. 2002;19:682–6.
47. Hadzic A, Vloka JD. Anterior approach to sciatic nerve block. In: Hadzic A, Vloka J, editors. Peripheral nerve blocks. New York, NY: McGraw-Hill; 2004.
48. Taboada M, Rodríguez J, Valiño C, Vazquez M, Laya A, Garea M, et al. A prospective, randomized comparison between the popliteal and subgluteal approaches for continuous sciatic nerve block with stimulating catheters. Anesth Analg. 2006 Jul;103(1):244–7.
49. di Benedetto P, Casati A, Bertini L. Continuous subgluteus sciatic nerve block after orthopedic foot and ankle surgery: comparison of two infusion techniques. Reg Anesth Pain Med. 2002;27(2):168–72.
50. Young DS, Cota A, Chaytor R. Continuous infragluteal sciatic nerve block for postoperative pain control after total ankle arthroplasty. Foot Ankle Spec. 2014;7(4):271–6.
51. Taboada M, Alvarez J, Cortés J, Rodríguez J, Rabanal S, Gude F, et al. The effects of three different approaches on the onset time of sciatic nerve blocks with 0.75% ropivacaine. Anesth Analg. 2004;98(1):242–7.
52. Yektaş A, Balkan B. Comparison of sciatic nerve block quality achieved using the anterior and posterior approaches: a randomised trial. BMC Anesthesiol. 2019;19:225.
53. Tammam TF. Ultrasound-guided sciatic nerve block: a comparison between four different infragluteal probe and needle alignment approaches. J Anesth. 2014;28:532–7.
54. Cao X, Zhao X, Xu J, Liu Z, Li Q. Ultrasound-guided technology versus neurostimulation for sciatic nerver block: a meta-analysis. Int J Clin Exp Med. 2015;8(1):273–80.
55. Danelli G, Ghisi D, Fanelli A, Ortu A, Moschini E, Berti M, et al. The effects of ultrasound guidance and neurostimulation the minimum effective anesthetic volume of mepivacaine 1.5% required to block the sciatic nerve using the subgluteal approach. Anesth Analg. 2009;109:1674–8.
56. Tantry TP, Kadam D, Shetty P, Bhandary S. Combined femoral and sciatic nerve blocks for lower limb anaesthesia in anticoagulated patients with severe cardiac valvular lesions. Indian J Anaesth. 2010;54(3):235–8.
57. Li J, Deng X, Jiang T. Combined femoral and sciatic nerve block versus femoral and local infiltration anesthesia for pain control after total knee arthroplasty: a meta-analysis of randomized controlled trials. J Orthop Surg Res. 2016;11:158.
58. Ota J, Sakura S, Hara K, Saito Y. Ultrasound-guided anterior approach to sciatic nerve block: a comparison with the posterior approach. Anesth Analg. 2009;108:660–5.
59. Barbero C, Fuzier R, Samii K. Anterior approach to the sciatic nerve block: adaptation to the patient's height. Anesth Analg. 2004;98:1785–8.
60. Singelyn FJ, Aye F, Gouverneur JM. Continuous popliteal sciatic nerve block: an original technique to provide postoperative analgesia after foot surgery. Anesth Analg. 1997;84:383–6.
61. Perlas A, Brull R, Chan VW, McCartney CJ, Nuica A, Abbas S. Ultrasound guidance improves the success of sciatic nerve block at the popliteal fossa. Reg Anesth Pain Med. 2008;33:259–65.
62. Danelli G, Fanelli A, Ghisi D, Moschini E, Rossi M, Ortu A, et al. Ultrasound vs nerve stimulation multiple injection technique for posterior popliteal sciatic nerve block. Anaesthesia. 2009;64:638–42.
63. Brull R, Macfarlane AJ, Parrington SJ, Koshkin A, Chan VW. Is circumferential injection advantageous for ultrasound-guided popliteal sciatic nerve block?: A proof-of-concept study. Reg Anesth Pain Med. 2011;36:266–70.

64. Buys MJ, Arndt CD, Vagh F, Hoard A, Gerstein N. Ultrasound-guided sciatic nerve block in the popliteal fossa using a lateral approach: onset time comparing separate tibial and common peroneal nerve injections versus injecting proximal to the bifurcation. Anesth Analg. 2010;110:635–7.
65. Prasad A, Perlas A, Ramlogan R, Brull R, Chan V. Ultrasound-guided popliteal block distal to sciatic nerve bifurcation shortens onset time: a prospective randomized double-blind study. Reg Anesth Pain Med. 2010;35:267–71.
66. Benzon HT, Kim C, Benzon HP, Silverstein ME, Jericho B, Prillaman K, et al. Correlation between evoked motor response of the sciatic nerve and sensory blockade. Anesthesiology. 1997;87:547–52.
67. Vloka JD, Hadzic A, April E, Thys DM. Division of the sciatic nerve in the popliteal fossa and its possible implications in the popliteal nerve blockade. Anesth Analg. 2001;92:215–7.
68. Monahan AM, Madison SJ, Loland VJ, Sztain JF, Bishop ML, Sandhu NS, et al. Continuous popliteal sciatic blocks: does varying perineural catheter location relative to the sciatic bifurcation influence block effects? A dual-center, randomized, subject-masked, controlled clinical trial. Anesth Analg. 2016;122(5):1689–95.
69. Lam NCK, Petersen TR, Gerstein NS, Yen T, Starr B, Mariano ER. A randomized clinical trial comparing the effectiveness of ultrasound guidance versus nerve stimulation for lateral popliteal-sciatic nerve blocks in obese patients. J Ultrasound Med. 2014;33(6):1057–63.
70. van Geffen GJ, van den Broek E, Braak GJ, Giele JL, Gielen MJ, Scheffer GJ. A prospective randomised controlled trial of ultrasound guided versus nerve stimulation guided distal sciatic nerve block at the popliteal fossa. Anaesth Intensive Care. 2009;37:32–7.
71. Ma HH, Chou TFA, Tsai SW, Chen CF, Wu PK, Chen WM. The efficacy and safety of continuous versus single-injection popliteal sciatic nerve block in outpatient foot and ankle surgery: a systematic review and meta-analysis. BMC Musculoskelet Disord. 2019;20(1):441.
72. Kerr DR, Kohan L. Local infiltration analgesia: a technique for the control of acute postoperative pain following knee and hip surgery: a case study of 325 patients. Acta Orthop. 2008;79:174–83.
73. Sankineani SR, Reddy ARC, Eachempati KK, Jangale A, Gurava Reddy AV. Comparison of adductor canal block and IPACK block (interspace between the popliteal artery and the capsule of the posterior knee) with adductor canal block alone after total knee arthroplasty: a prospective control trial on pain and knee function in immediate postoperative period. Eur J Orthop Surg Traumatol. 2018;28:1391–5.
74. Soares LG, Brull R, Chan VW. Teaching an old block a new trick: ultrasound-guided posterior tibial nerve block. Acta Anaesthesiol Scand. 2008;52:446–7.
75. Redborg KE, Sites BD, Chinn CD, Gallagher JD, Ball PA, Antonakakis JG, et al. Ultrasound improves the success rate of a sural nerve block at the ankle. Reg Anesth Pain Med. 2009;34:24–8.
76. Doty R Jr, Sukhani R, Kendall MC, Yaghmour E, Nader A, Brodskaia A, Kataria TC, McCarthy R. Evaluation of a proximal block site and the use of nerve-stimulator-guided needle placement for posterior tibial nerve block. Anesth Analg. 2006;103:1300–5.

Truncal Blocks

4

Arunangshu Chakraborty, Rakhi Khemka, and Amit Dikshit

4.1 Introduction

The use of ultrasound in regional anaesthesia was initially limited to peripheral nerve blocks until Hebbard et al. [1] described the ultrasound-guided transversus abdominis plane (TAP) block.

The unique feature of the ultrasound-guided truncal blocks is that in all of these techniques, in contrast to peripheral nerve blocks no nerve or plexus need to be identified. The local anaesthetic (LA) is injected in a particular muscle plane, in which the injectate spreads and reaches the intended nerves. This simple mechanism has made the delivery of nerve blocks easy and versatile.

The truncal blocks can be broadly divided into blocks in the abdominal wall, blocks in the chest wall and blocks in the back (Table 4.1).

4.2 Blocks in the Anterior Abdominal Wall

4.2.1 Transversus Abdominis Plane (TAP) Block

The anterior branch of intercostal nerves $T_{7\text{-}12}$, that innervate the anterior abdominal wall along with the anterior rami of first lumbar spinal nerve (L_1) travel in the plane between the internal oblique (IOM) and transversus abdominis muscles (TAM) [2]. The technique aims to inject 15–20 mL LA in the plane between these muscles (Fig. 4.1). The landmark-based technique was first described by Dr. Rafi [3]. The technique consisted of eliciting two 'pops' or loss of resistance by a blunt-tipped

A. Chakraborty (✉)
Department of Anaesthesia, CC and Pain, Tata Medical Center, Kolkata, India

R. Khemka
Tata Medical Center, Kolkata, India

A. Dikshit
Rubi Hall Clinic, Pune, India

A. Chakraborty (ed.), *Blockmate*, https://doi.org/10.1007/978-981-15-9202-7_4

Table 4.1 Types of truncal blocks

Blocks in the abdominal wall	Blocks in the chest wall	Blocks in the back
1. Transversus abdominis plane (TAP) block 2. Rectus sheath block 3. Ilioinguinal and iliohypogastric block 4. Quadratus lumborum block A. QLB 1 B. QLB 2 C. QLB 3 D. Lumbar interfascial triangle (LIFT) block	1. Pectoral nerves block (Pecs-I and II) 2. Serratus anterior plane (SAP) block 3. Intercostal nerve block 4. Interpleural block	1. Erector Spinae Plane block—Thoracic, lumbar, sacral 2. Thoracolumbar interfascial plane (TLIP) block 3. Thoracic paravertebral block

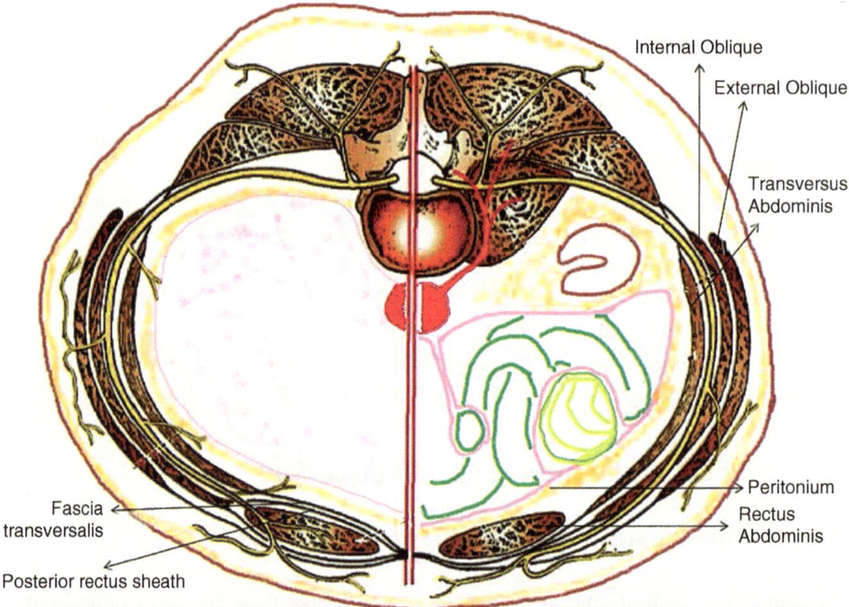

Fig. 4.1 Muscles of abdominal wall and the course of the nerves

needle entering perpendicularly at the lumbar triangle of Petit. For midline surgeries, the block has to be repeated on both sides. TAP block is the easiest to learn and the most widely practiced truncal block.

There are four described approaches of TAP block

1. *Posterior TAP:* Injection in the lumbar triangle of Petit. Usually employed in the landmark-based technique [4–7]. Here the drug is injected between the fascia transversalis and the internal oblique muscle. This technique is considered the precursor of the quadratus lumborum block.

2. *Lateral TAP:* LA is injected in the neurovascular plane between the IOM and TAM with the ultrasound transducer (UST) placed transversely in the anterior axillary line, above the iliac crest [6, 7] (Fig. 4.2).
3. *Anterior TAP:* Ultrasound transducer is held transversely in the mid clavicular line and scanned laterally till the three abdominal muscles are seen. The needle is inserted from medial to lateral and the drug deposited in the TAP plane (Fig. 4.3).

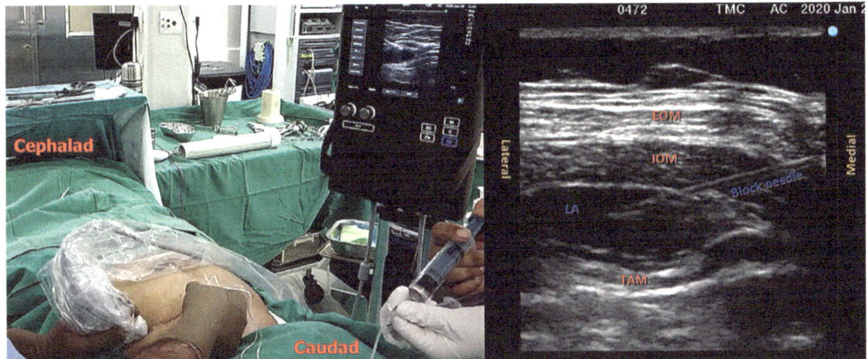

Fig. 4.2 Lateral TAP block: Note the patient position and transducer orientation. *EOM* external oblique muscle, *IOM* internal oblique muscle, *TAM* transversus abdominis muscle, *LA* local anaesthetic

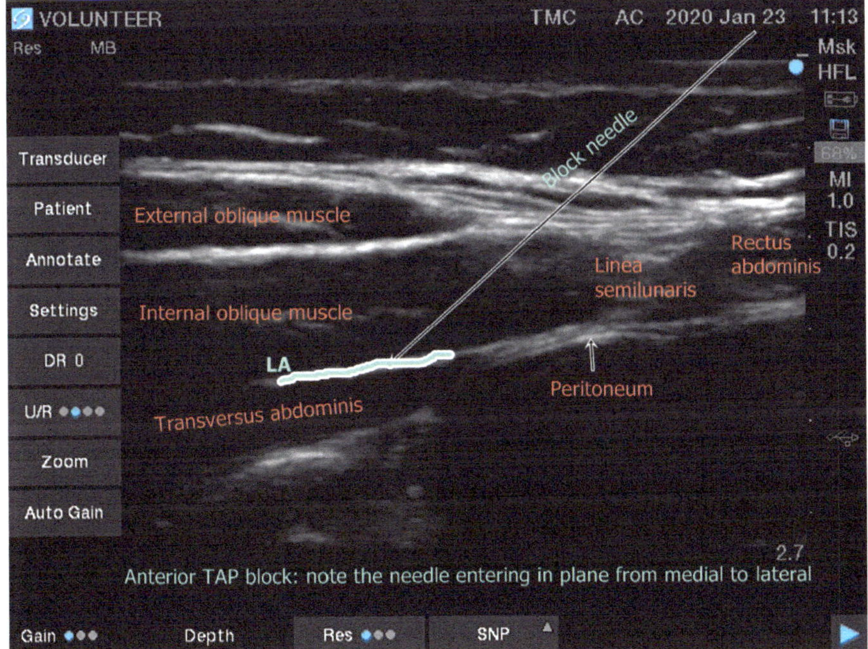

Fig. 4.3 Anterior TAP: Note the local anaesthetic (LA) is deposited between TA and IO muscles

4. *Oblique subcostal TAP:* Injection in the subcostal area, LA is injected between the posterior rectus sheath and TAM [8] (Fig. 4.4a, b).

Oblique subcostal TAP (OSTAP) is also called 'upper TAP' block. The term 'Dual TAP' means the administration of TAP block in both 'lower', i.e. lateral approach and 'upper' area [9, 10]. Bilateral administration of dual TAP block (BDTAP) is required to provide complete analgesia to the anterior abdominal wall. This method is also known as 'four quadrant' TAP block [11].

Ultrasound Technique Ultrasound-guided TAP block is considered as a 'basic level' skill block. The patient is placed supine, however a lateral position may be helpful in an obese patient [12]. A Linear UST with frequency between 10 and 18 MHz with depth setting adjusted between 3 and 5 cm (depending upon the amount of adipose tissue) is placed transversely across the abdomen above the iliac crest at the anterior axillary line. External oblique (EOM), IOM and TAM (superfi-

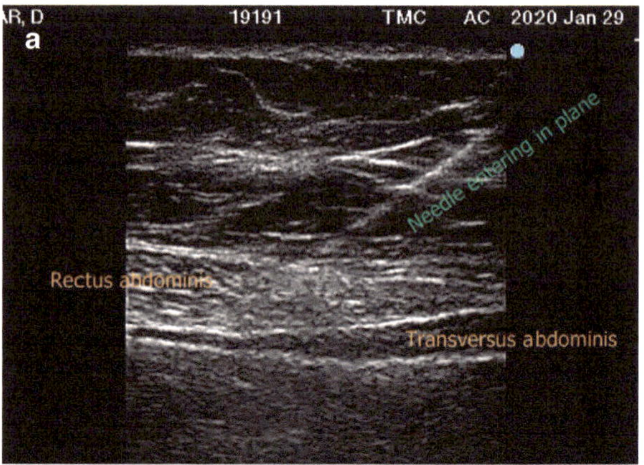

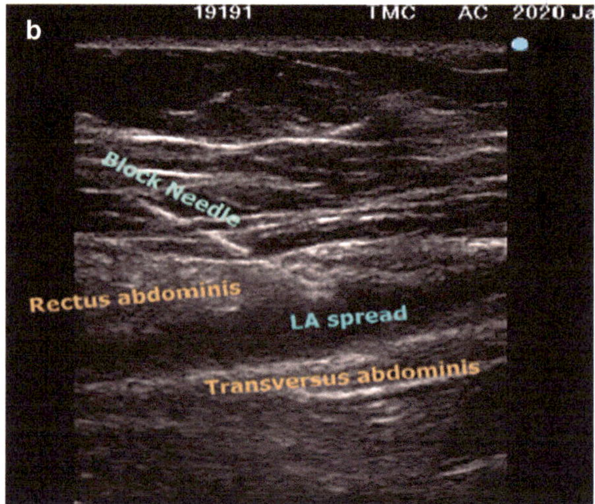

Fig. 4.4 (**a**) OSTAP: Note the needle inserting in plane. (**b**) OSTAP: Note the LA spread

cial to deep) can be easily identified below the adipose tissue and IOM is usually the most prominent muscle among the three. The peritoneal cavity lies deep to the TAM and can be identified by the movement of the bowel loops. If it is difficult to identify all the three layers then the UST should be placed at the midline and rectus abdominis muscle (RAM) is identified and the UST is moved laterally where RAM tapers and ends in the linea semilunaris and the obliques begin. The UST is then moved laterally to a point where the three muscles can be clearly demarcated and the needle is introduced. A 100 mm 20G/22G blunt-tipped needle is chosen and introduced from anterior to posterior or medial to the lateral direction. The aim is to inject 15–20 mL LA in the plane between the IOM and TAM muscles. Accurate placement of the needle tip may be facilitated by injection of a small amount of fluid (1–2 mL of saline or local anaesthetic) to 'hydro dissect' the appropriate plane. The correct placement of the injectate is confirmed by seeing the spindle-shaped hypoechoic fluid pocket in the space lined by the hyperechoic fascia of the IOM and the TAM after the injection.

For the *oblique subcostal* TAP block, the UST is placed just below the costal margin close to the midline and RAM is identified. In the subcostal area, TAM lies deep to the rectus muscle. The block needle is then introduced into the plane between the posterior rectus sheath (PRS) and TAM. The Block needle is gradually advanced laterally through hydrodissection till we can see EOM and IOM along the lateral border of the rectus. Total of 20–25 mL of anaesthetic solution is given along the line between the xiphoid process and iliac crest. OSTAP is considered an 'advanced level' block.

Indications

Analgesia for laparoscopic surgeries, hysterectomies, lower segment caesarean section (LSCS), herniorrhaphy, etc.

An 'upper' TAP block is more effective in upper abdominal surgeries, while pain relief for sub umbilical surgeries is well addressed by 'lower' TAP block. Four quadrant TAP block has been used for postoperative analgesia in laparotomies using a larger incision (Fig. 4.5).

Complications Complications such as intraperitoneal injection, liver trauma and catheter breakage have been reported with TAP block, however; with the use of ultrasound the incidence of complications has reduced considerably.

Blockmate Pearls

- TAP block is considered a learner's/beginner's block. The landmarks are easy to identify and there is minimal risk of complications.
- Bilateral TAP can be used for analgesia after LSCS.
- Although labelled as beginners block, needle visualization can be challenging, particularly in obese patients. The use of echogenic needles (e.g. Sonoplex, Pajunk, Geisingen, Germany) helps in needle imaging.
- The golden principles for deeper blocks are

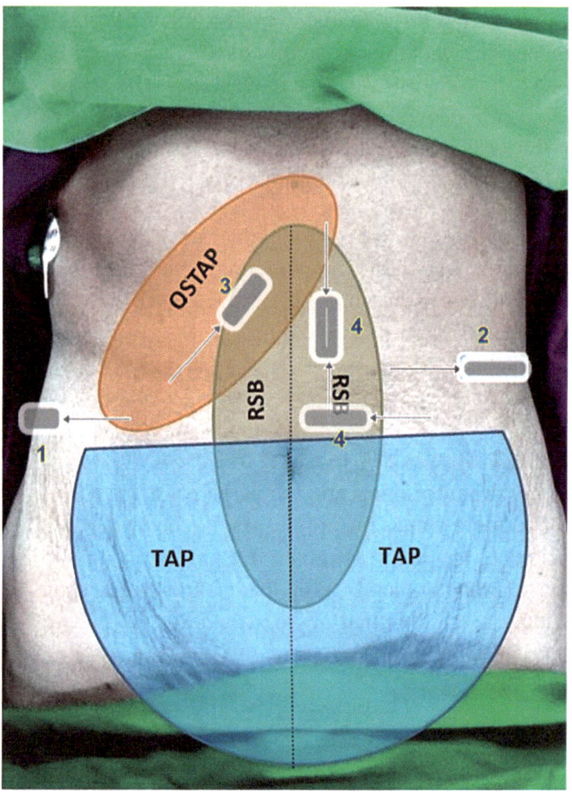

Fig. 4.5 Probe position, needle trajectory and sensory distribution of anterior abdominal wall blocks. The grey box represents the probe position and the arrow the block needle. (1) Lateral TAP, (2) anterior TAP, (3) OSTAP and (4) RSB. The shaded areas represent the extent of sensory effect of the blocks as mentioned

1. Use low-frequency curvilinear transducer and.
2. Enter the skin 2–3 cm away from the lateral edge of the transducer so that the needle trajectory lies at a more acute angle to the US beam and reflect more US and become brightly visible in the ultrasound.

4.2.2 Rectus Sheath Block

The rectus sheath block (RSB) was first described in 1899 and was initially used for the purpose of abdominal wall muscle relaxation during laparotomy before the introduction of neuromuscular block. Now, it is used for analgesia after umbilical or incisional hernia repairs and other midline surgical incisions. The aim is to block the terminal branches of the 9–11th intercostal nerves which run in between IOM and TAM to penetrate the posterior wall of RAM and end in an anterior cutaneous branch supplying the skin of the umbilical area [13]. A catheter can be placed for continuous infusion of LA [14].

Ultrasound Technique A high-frequency linear array UST is held transversely over the rectus abdominis muscle (RAM), which can be easily identified by its spindle-like shape on the transverse section. A 22G Tuohy needle is inserted into the plane between RAM and the posterior rectus sheath (PRS) and 10–15 mL of LA is injected. A catheter may be placed for a continuous block. For inserting the catheter, the UST is rotated by 90° and a plane is created between RAM and PRS by hydrodissection. The catheter is advanced 5–6 cm into space. Bilateral catheter is required for a midline surgery (Fig. 4.6a, b).

Indications Post-operative analgesia for umbilical hernia repair and other umbilical surgery.

Transducer position: transverse on the abdomen, immediately lateral to the umbilicus.

Complications Wound infection and catheter migration to intraperitoneal space are known complications of RSB. The ultrasound-guided technique is remarkably safe.

Blockmate Pearls

- RSB is considered a learner's/beginner's block. The landmarks are easy to identify and there is minimal risk of complications.

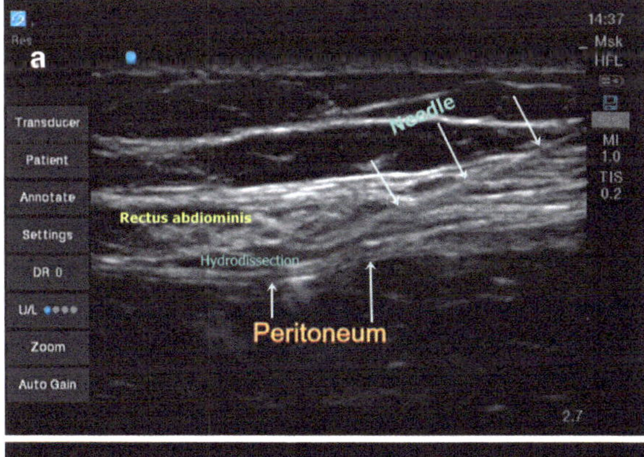

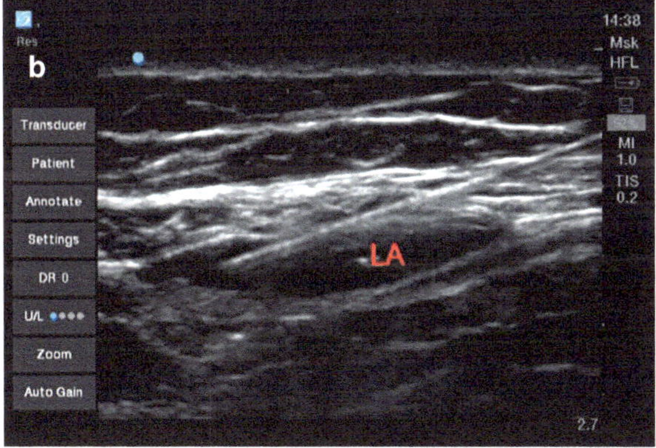

Fig. 4.6 (**a**) Rectus sheath block: Note the needle is inserted in plane, from lateral to medial direction, US transducer being held in a transverse orientation. (**b**) Rectus sheath block: Note the local anaesthetic (LA) has been injected between the rectus abdominis muscle and its posterior sheath

Table 4.2 Variations of the quadratus lumborum block (QLB)

Block	Patient position	Ultrasound technique	Injection endpoint
QLB1	Supine or lateral	Transducer: linear or curvilinear Needle approach: in plane, lateral to medial	Lateral edge of the QLB muscle, below the fascia transversalis
QLB2	Lateral or prone	Transducer: linear or curvilinear Needle approach: in plane, lateral to medial	Plane between erector spinae muscle and QLB
QLB3 also called the transmuscular QLB (Fig. 4.7)	Lateral or prone	Transducer: curvilinear Needle approach: in plane, posterior to anterior, the transducer placed over the L4 spine to obtain the 'shamrock' image, With the psoas muscle anteriorly, the erector spinae muscle posteriorly and QL attached to the apex of the transverse process, a recognizable pattern of a shamrock with three leaves can be seen [16]	Plane between QLB and psoas major muscle
Lumbar interfascial triangle (LIFT) block	Lateral or prone	Transducer: linear or curvilinear Needle approach: in plane, lateral to medial or out of plane. Lumbar interfascial triangle is imaged as a triangular space bound by latissimus dorsi muscle (roof), medially the lateral edge of erector spinae muscle, base by posterior surface of QLB	Lumbar interfascial triangle

- It is a very versatile block. The transducer can be held transversely or longitudinally. Accordingly, needle is inserted from lateral to medial or from cephalad to caudal direction.
- For catheter placement the longitudinal approach is helpful.
- RSB being a superficial block, can be even performed with a hypodermic needle. Blunting the needle end helps in appreciation of loss of resistance when the muscle is pierced.

4.2.3 Quadratus Lumborum Block

Quadratus lumborum block (QLB) is a posterior extension of the transversus abdominis plane block. First described by Dr. Blanco [15], it was later modified by Sauter et al. [16]. Recent developments have elaborated this technique into four distinct techniques which are QLB 1, 2, 3 and the lumbar interfascial triangle (LIFT) block, each having a different approach and injection endpoint (Table 4.2). Being a deeper block, difficulty wise they have been categorized as moderate to advanced level (Figs. 4.8 and 4.9).

All of the blocks can be used as a single shot or a catheter can be inserted for continuous infusion.

Imaging studies have shown that the injected local anaesthetic in QLB3 reaches the paravertebral space [17, 18]. Thus QLB has been claimed to cause better

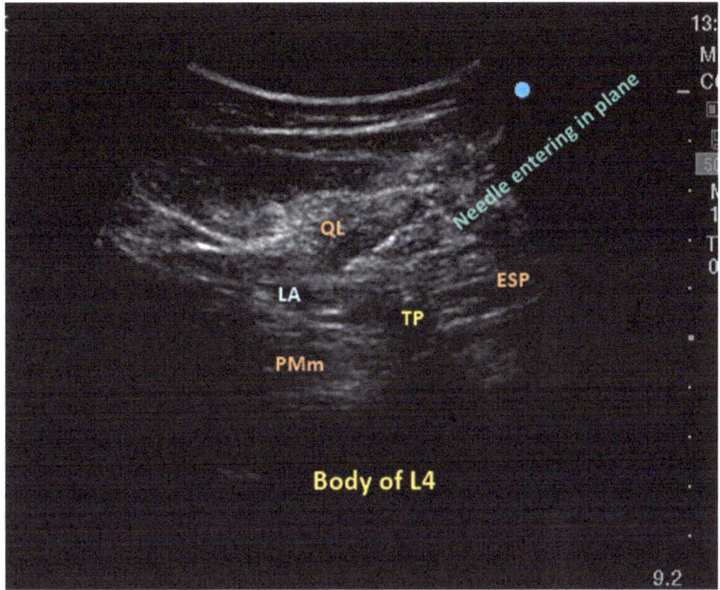

Fig. 4.7 Transmuscular QL (QL3): Note the 'shamrock sign'—the transverse process (TP) of the fourth lumbar vertebra (L4) forming the stock of the 'shamrock', while the erector spinae (ESP), quadratus lumborum (QL) and psoas major muscle (PMm) forms the three petals. The local anaesthetic (LA) is deposited in the plane between QL and PMm

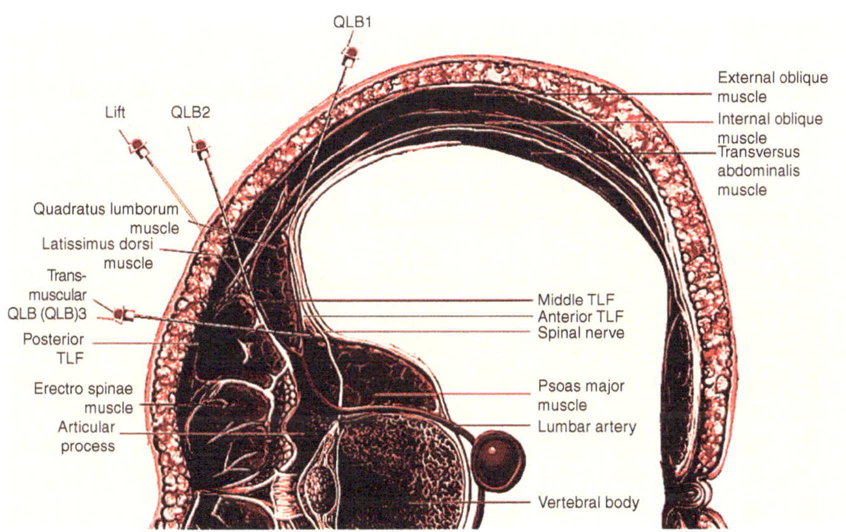

Fig 4.8 Variations of Quadratus lumborum block: QLB 1, 2, 3 and LIFT

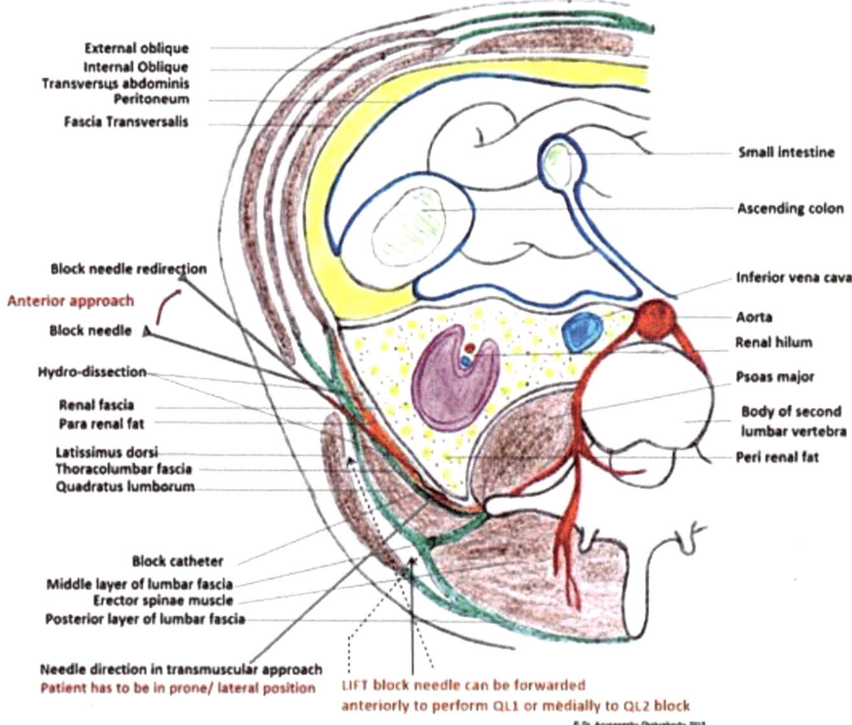

Fig. 4.9 Anatomical basis of QL blocks. Note how the LIFT block can be extended laterally as QL1 and medially as QL2 blocks

analgesia than TAP block as it not only provides analgesia to the anterior abdominal wall, it blocks visceral pain too.

An *anterior approach* [19] has been described in paediatric patients, where a *linear* UST is held transversely in the posterior axillary line, and LA is injected in the plane between the anterior surface of the quadratus lumborum muscle and the thoracolumbar fascia.

The lumbar plexus lying in the psoas major muscle is in near vicinity of the QLB area of injection, and as such can be blocked to some extent. Some clinical reports suggest its use in hip surgeries.

QL1 block can be performed with a curvilinear UST with the patient in supine position also where the UST is held transversely lateral to the mid clavicular line and the needle enters from medial to the lateral direction. For the beginners however, the first approach should be with the patient in the lateral position and the needle entering from the posterior to the anterior direction (Fig. 5.5).

LIFT block (Fig. 4.10) is a superficial block that can be performed using a linear or a curvilinear UST. Out of plane LIFT block can be performed even with a standard hypodermic needle in a lean patient. The LIFT block can be easily converted to a QL1 in the same way by hydrodissecting the plane and advancing the needle anteriorly (Fig. 4.11).

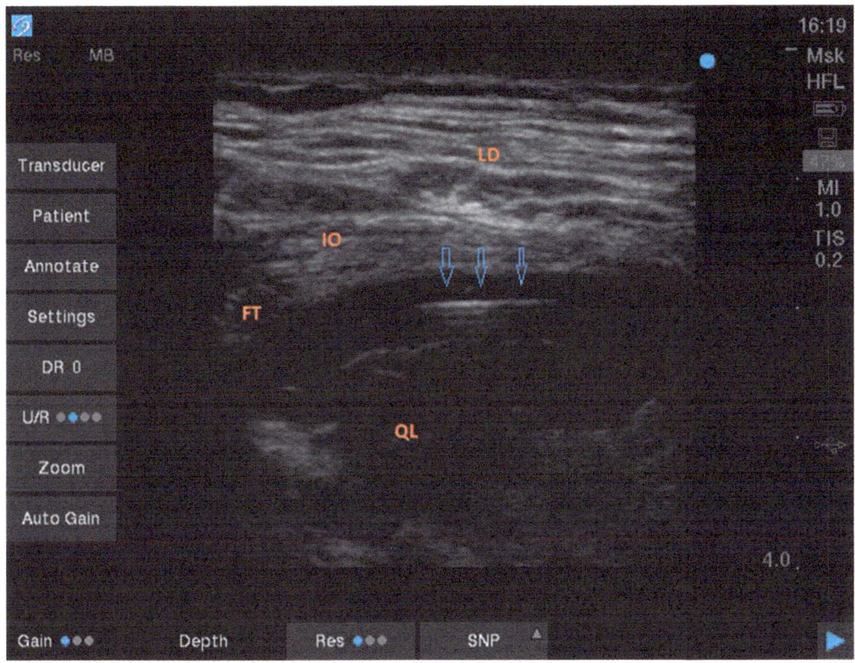

Fig. 4.10 Performing the QL1 block with a linear UST

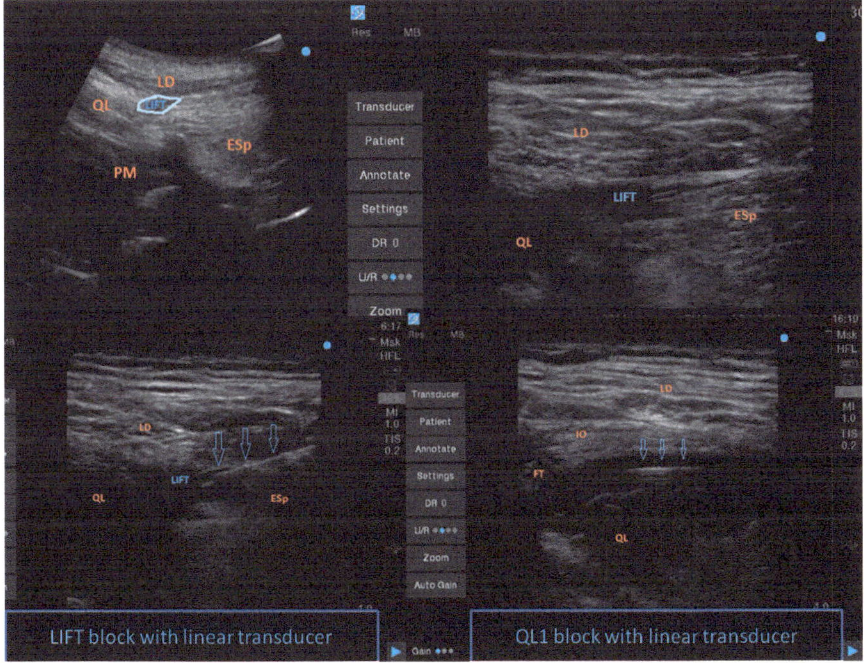

Fig. 4.11 Top left: LIFT scanning with a curvilinear UST, Top right: LIFT scanning with a linear UST, Bottom left: LIFT block with a linear UST, Bottom right: extension of LIFT into QL1 by anterior hydrodissection and needle advancement

Indications

- QLB cannot be employed for surgical anaesthesia but it provides post-operative analgesia. It is best employed as part of a multimodal analgesia regimen. Pre-emptive QLB in conjunction with general anaesthesia can reduce the intraoperative analgesic requirement.
- Unilateral QLB can be used to provide post-operative analgesia in unilateral abdominal surgeries, such as nephrectomy.
- Bilateral QLB can be employed for a wide variety of lower abdominal surgeries starting from the low segment caesarean section (LSCS) to colorectal operations to provide post-operative analgesia.

Complications No complications have been reported so far with this block, however; catheter migration to retroperitoneal space is a concern.

Blockmate Pearls

- QL1 and LIFT are technically easier to perform.
- QL3 is a deep block, graded as advanced. Only experienced users should attempt.
- Needle imaging is difficult in deeper blocks, hence the risk of inadvertent injury more. It is prudent to avoid QL3 in coagulopathic patients.

4.2.4 Ilioinguinal and Iliohypogastric (Hernia Block)

The iliohypogastric (IHN) and ilioinguinal (IIN) nerves arise from the first lumbar nerve and emerge from the upper part of the lateral border of the psoas major muscle. IIN is the smaller of the two and travels caudal to IHN. As the lateral cutaneous branch of IHN may pierce the internal and external oblique muscles immediately above the iliac crest, the nerves should be blocked as proximal as possible i.e. just above the iliac crest so these cutaneous branches are not spared.

Field block for inguinal hernia surgery has been administered since the 1980s [20–23].

Studies indicate that the ultrasound-guided TAP block approach is superior to landmark-based approaches of II and IH block [24–27]. This block has been used extensively in pediatric anaesthesia practice [28].

Ultrasound Technique The patient is placed supine and the UST (linear) is placed obliquely just above the iliac crest along the line joining the anterior superior iliac spine and umbilicus [23, 24]. A 5–8 cm 22G needle is inserted in plane. LA is deposited in the same plane as that of TAP block, i.e. between the IOM and TAM muscles. LA is injected per side about 10–15 mL. The correct placement of the needle is identified by the expansion of the space lined by the hyperechoic fascia of IOM and TAM after the injection (Figs. 4.12 and 4.13).

Indications Anaesthesia and post-operative analgesia for inguinal hernia repair and other inguinal surgery; analgesia following suprapubic incision.

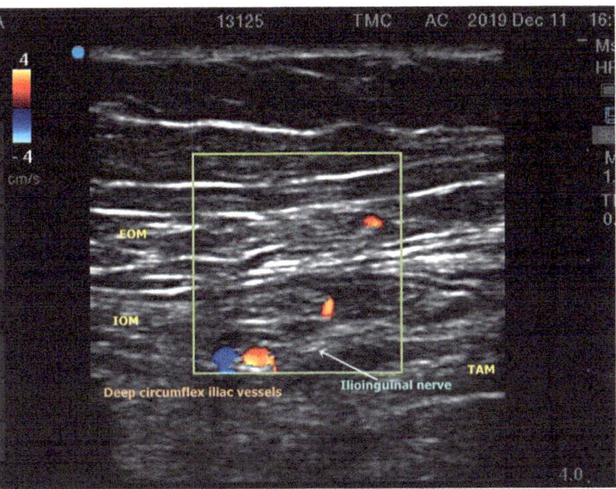

Fig. 4.12 Ilioinguinal and iliohypogastric nerve block: the deep circumflex vessels are imaged with colour doppler, the ilioinguinal nerve lies close. *EOM* external oblique muscle, *IOM* internal oblique muscle, *TAM* transversus abdominis muscle

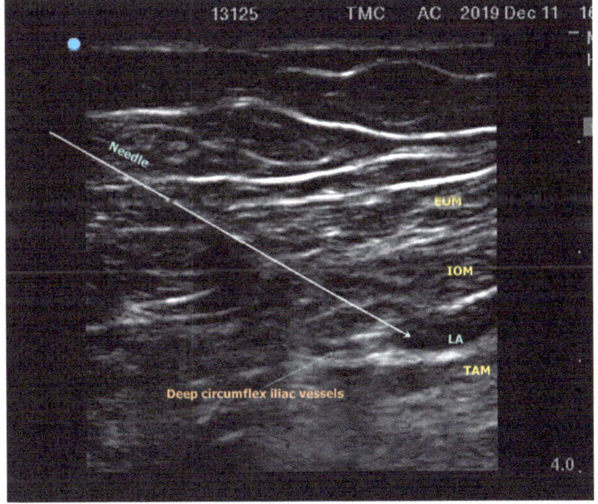

Fig. 4.13 Local anaesthetic (LA) is injected after identification of the plane with hydrodissection

Complications Intraperitoneal injection and femoral nerve block are known complications.

4.2.5 Spermatic Cord Block or Genitofemoral Nerve Block

The spermatic cord is bound by the external spermatic fascia (derived from external oblique aponeurosis, the cremasteric muscle and its fascia (derived from internal oblique) and internal spermatic fascia, which is the continuation of fascia transversalis. It contains vas deferens, pampiniform (venous) plexus, testicular artery and lymphatics. The genitofemoral nerve lies between the external and internal spermatic fascia, adjacent to the cremasteric muscle layer.

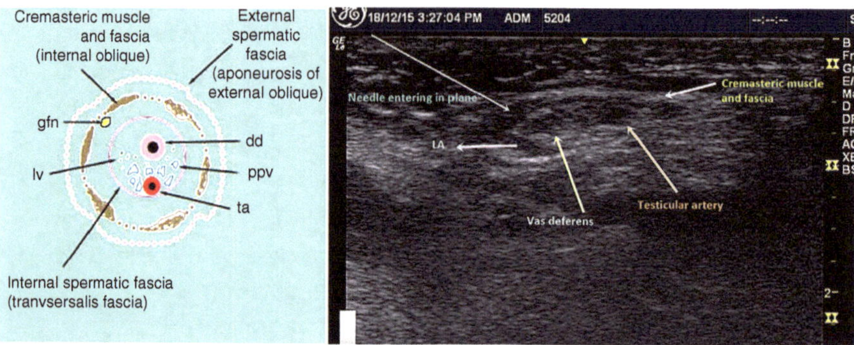

Fig. 4.14 Left: Cross-sectional anatomy of spermatic cord. *dd* ductus (vas) deferens, *ppv* pampiniform venous plexus, *ta* testicular artery, *gfn* genitofemoral nerve, *lv* lymph vessels; Right: US image of spermatic cord block: Note the spermatic fascia covering the testicular artery and vas deferens

With ultrasound it is easy to find out the spermatic cord and its contents. A high-frequency linear UST is used to image and identify the spermatic cord as an oval structure lying medial and superficial to the femoral artery [29]. The scout scan can start from the symphysis pubis and then moved laterally till the cord is imaged. In lean patients the cord is palpable, making placement of the UST easier. Block can be attempted below or at the level of inguinal ligament. Colour doppler can point out the vessels. Care must be taken to avoid the blood vessels in close vicinity [30, 31]. The advantage of the ultrasound technique over landmark-based technique lies in the ability to avoid damage to vascular structures and resulting hematoma. An ultrasound-guided spermatic cord block can produce analgesia lasting 8–16 h (Fig. 4.14).

Indications Scrotal surgeries, chronic pain in the genitofemoral nerve area [29].

Complications Vascular trauma is apprehended but with the use of ultrasound, the block is safer.

Blockmate Pearls

- Spermatic cord block can be employed for orchidectomies, in conjunction with general anaesthesia or SAB for post-operative analgesia.

4.3 Blocks in the Chest Wall

The chest wall is innervated by the lateral intercostal nerves, which are branches of the anterior rami of spinal nerves of thoracic division 2nd to 12th. While the cutaneous innervation is through the intercostal nerves, the chest wall muscles, pectoralis major and minor are supplied by the lateral and medial pectoral nerves, which originate from the brachial plexus. Other major chest wall muscles such as serratus anterior (long thoracic nerve—arising from the upper trunk of the brachial plexus) and latissimus dorsi (thoracodorsal nerve—arising from the posterior cord of the brachial plexus) are also supplied by the brachial plexus and generally lie in the muscle plane that can be breached by the Pecs block. A thoracic paravertebral block can provide cutaneous analgesia, but cannot provide analgesia to the areas supplied by the pectoral nerves. The pectoral nerves block was designed to block the said nerves. Along with the pectoral nerves, by virtue of diffusion along the muscle plane, the LA injected in a 'Pecs' block also reaches the intercostal nerves, thereby providing cutaneous analgesia as well.

4.3.1 The Pecs Block

The Lateral Pectoral Nerve (LPN) and the Medial Pectoral nerve (MPN) are branches of the brachial plexus that innervate pectoral muscles. LPN arises from the lateral cord of the brachial plexus, and from the roots of fifth–seventh cervical nerves. MPN originates from the medial cord of the brachial plexus from roots C_8 and T_1 [32]. LPN pierces the coracoclavicular fascia, and is distributed to the deep surface of the Pectoralis major and innervates its clavicular head. LPN provides sensory innervation to acromioclavicular joint, subacromial bursa, periosteum of the clavicle and anterior articular capsule of the shoulder joint and costoclavicular ligaments [33]. MPN enters the deep surface of the Pectoralis minor, where it supplies the muscle. Two or three of its branches pierce the muscle and end in the Pectoralis major and innervate its costal head. MPN gives sensory innervation to the inferolateral part of the pectoralis major, the ventral aspect of the arm and the chest wall near the armpit along with the intercostobrachial nerve (Fig. 4.15).

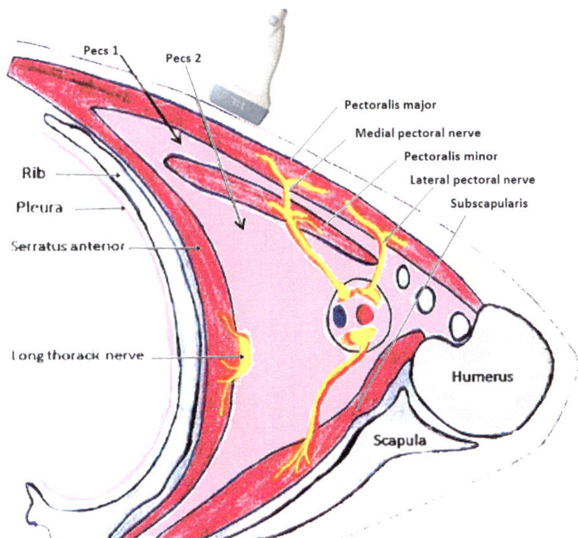

Fig. 4.15 Anatomy of pecs block

Pecs-1 The Pec 1 block is an interfascial plane block that aims to block the lateral and medial pectoral nerves. Local anaesthetic about 10–15 mL is injected between the pectoralis major (PMm) and minor (Pmm) muscles. The block is safely and reliably done under US guidance with the help of high resolution linear UST (Fig. 4.16).

Indications Breast surgeries such as lumpectomy, breast expander/prosthesis [34].

Pec 2 In Pec 2 block 20 mL of local anaesthetic is injected between the lateral edge of the pectoralis minor muscle and the serratus muscle at the level of the third rib. The aim is to block the lateral rami of intercostal nerves and the long thoracic nerve. This block is useful for most of the breast surgeries including axillary dissections [35, 36].

Technique
For the pectoral blocks the patient is placed supine and a linear high-frequency UST is used. Depth is usually set at 3–5 cm.

Pec 1 The UST is either held in a sagittal plane (same as in infraclavicular brachial plexus block) as described by Blanco [34] or is placed below the lateral one third of the clavicle transverse to the axis of the body [36]. The needle is directed from superomedial to inferolateral direction in both the approaches. Cranially we can see the clavicle and below it we can see pectoralis major (superficial) and pectoralis minor (deep). Deep to the muscles, we can see the axillary artery and the vein. If a rib is visualized it is usually the second rib and the pleura can be seen as a bright hyper echoic line beneath it. For pecs-1 block, the 5–8 cm 22G block needle is inserted and advanced in plane to the UST from cranial to caudal direction and 10 mL of LA solution is injected between the two muscle layers.

Pec 2 Block The UST is moved caudally from the Pecs 1 position till the third and the fourth ribs are visualized. The UST is then rotated 90° so that it lies *transversely* and moves laterally towards the anterior axillary line keeping the third rib at the centre so that the lateral border of pectoralis minor is identified. Serratus anterior muscle is seen deeper to the pectoralis minor lying on top of the third rib. The needle

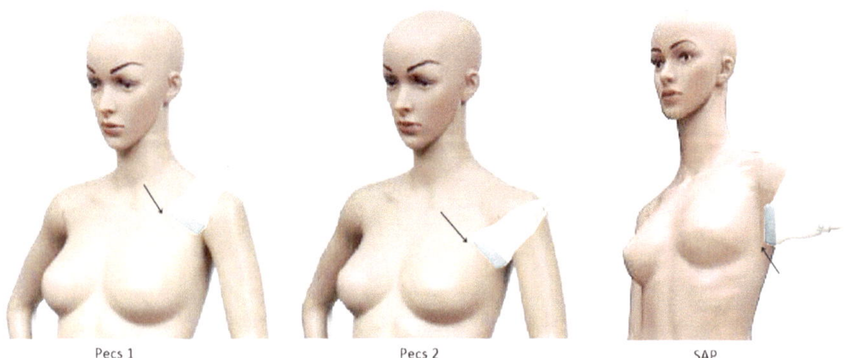

Fig. 4.16 Probe position for Pec 1, Pec 2 and SAP blocks

is advanced from medial to lateral side parallel to the US beam and 20 mL of LA solution is injected in the plane between pectoralis minor and serratus anterior.

In the original Pecs 2 technique, two-needle passes were described. Recently a single injection technique has been described, which has been called '*Combipecs*' [37]. As the name suggests, the technique combines the two injections of Pecs 2 into 1. The UST is held in the anterior axillary line over the third rib, centred over a point where all the three muscle layers (PMn, Pmm and SA) can be imaged. The block needle is inserted in plane and 15–20 mL LA is injected in the plane between Pmm and SA. While withdrawing, hydrodissection is done to confirm needle placement in the plane between PMm and Pmm. Another 10 mL LA is injected here. This technique (Fig. 4.17) reduces time required for the block as well as reduces patient discomfort as only a single needle pass is required.

Indications

- Pecs 1 can be used for analgesia for superficial anterior chest wall procedures such as insertion of pacemaker, chemoport, etc.
- Pecs 2 and Combipecs can be used for breast surgery with axillary dissection, breast implant insertion, etc.

Complications No complications have been reported so far, but pneumothorax and trauma to vessels such as the thoracodorsal artery are concerns with these techniques.

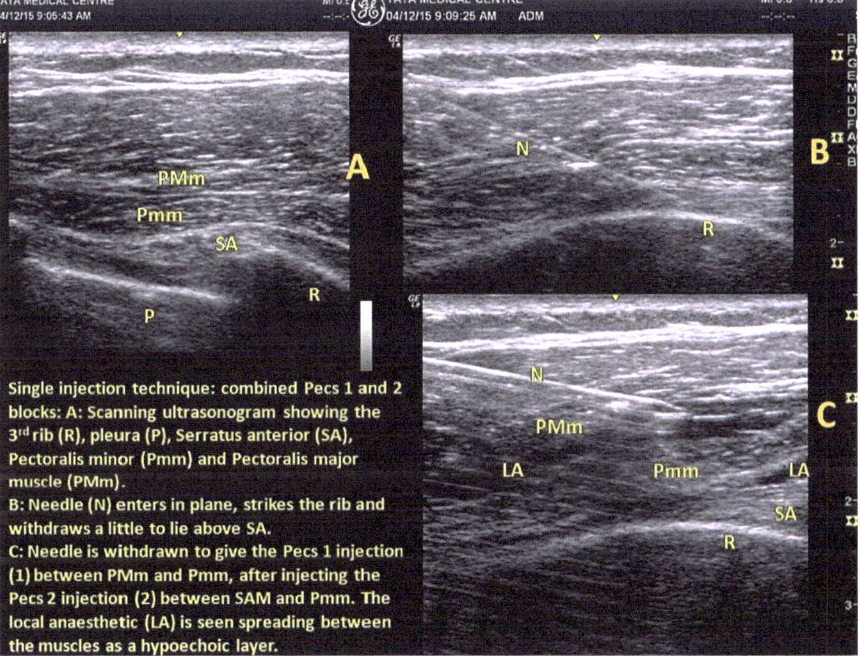

Fig. 4.17 The combipecs technique

Blockmate Pearls

- The upper part of the chest wall from the clavicle till the second rib receives cutaneous innervation from supraclavicular nerves which arise from the cervical nerve roots 3–5. For analgesia of this part a 'clavipectoral fascia block' can be used. In simpler terms, 5–10 mL LA infiltration over the middle third of the clavicle can block these nerves which traverse in the subcutaneous plane.
- A superficial cervical plexus blockade can augment the Pecs 2 block for an upper frontal thoracic wall surgery.
- The medial/parasternal chest wall is innervated by anterior cutaneous branches of the intercostal nerves. They can be blocked by a pecto-intercostal fascial block where LA is deposited between PMm and external intercostal muscle in the parasternal area. The needle is inserted from medial to lateral targeting the second, third and fourth costal cartilage.

4.3.2 Serratus Anterior Plane Block (SAP)

The Serratus anterior plane (SAP) block is a recently described regional block, designed to block the thoracic intercostal nerves along with the thoracodorsal and the long thoracic nerves. It aims to provide analgesia to the anterolateral and part of the posterior side of the chest wall, as an alternative to epidural and paravertebral blocks. SAP block was described in healthy volunteers without clinical validation. The sensory paresthesia was described in dermatomes from $T_{2\text{-}9}$. In this block, the injectate is administered either superficial or deep to the serratus anterior muscle, and the difference is only the duration of the block. The duration of the block was found to be doubled if the LA solution was injected superficial to the SA muscle. Serratus plane block is a variation of Pecs-2; only the needle is placed in more caudally and

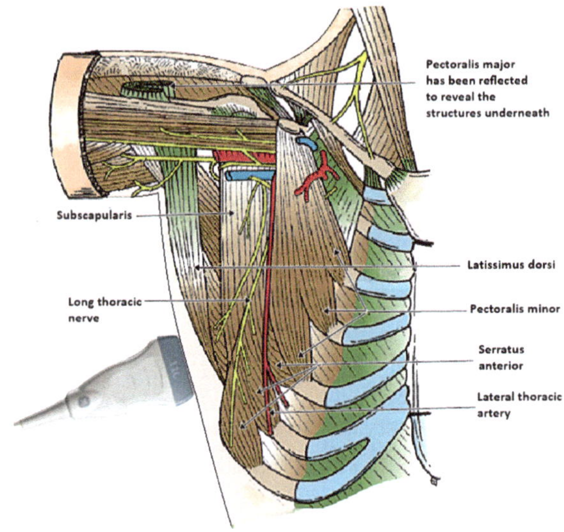

Fig. 4.18 Anatomy of SAP block

posteriorly compared to Pecs-2 block (Fig. 4.18). The needle is advanced 'in plane' from caudal to cranial approach at the level of midaxillary line [37, 38].

Technique This block is usually performed in lateral or sitting decubitus. The UST is moved caudally (from Pec 2 position) and laterally towards the mid axillary line counting the ribs and serratus anterior muscle is identified as a thin sheet lying above the ribs. Keeping the fifth rib in the middle of the ultrasound screen, the block needle is inserted in a plane from anteromedial to posterolateral direction. LA solution about 20 mL is injected in the mid axillary line at the level of the fifth rib either superficial or deep to the serratus anterior (Figs. 4.19 and 4.20).

To prevent inadvertent pneumothorax it is important to aim the needle towards the rib. The Pecs-2 and the SAP block are considered 'advanced level' skill blocks because of the vicinity of crucial structures and demanding technique.

Indications SAP produces analgesia of the hemithorax. A few clinical reports are available about its efficacy for post-op analgesia [39].

Complications No complications have been reported so far, but pneumothorax is a concern.

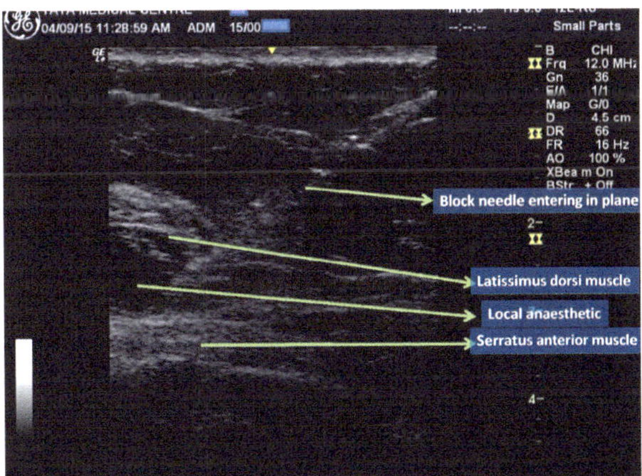

Fig. 4.19 SAP block: Note the LA being administered between the Latissimus dorsi and the serratus anterior muscles

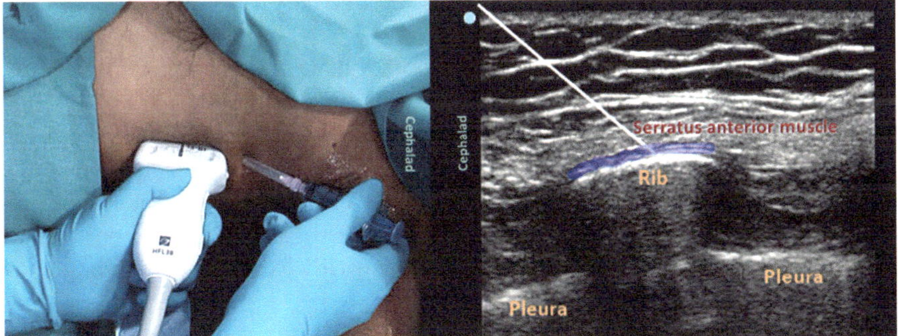

Fig. 4.20 SAP block between the serratus anterior muscle and the rib. Note the probe position and needle advancement in plane

Blockmate Pearls

- SAP block is useful for analgesia for multiple rib fractures. In contrast to intercostal blocks, a single injection of 10–15 mL of LA is adequate to cover 3–4 rib spaces.

4.3.3 Intercostal Nerves Block

Anatomy The intercostal nerves arise from the ventral rami of the thoracic spinal nerve. They are mixed nerves containing both sensory and motor fibres. The collateral branch of the intercostal nerve runs along the upper border of the rib below. It gives motor innervations to the intercostal muscles, latissimus dorsi, serratus anterior and the abdominal wall muscles and sensory innervations to the pleura, peritoneum, anterior and lateral chest and abdominal walls.

The intercostal block produces a stretch of band like anaesthesia along the chosen plane [40, 41].

Indications For providing surgical anaesthesia for thoracic and upper abdominal procedures and for pain management in case of chest trauma, flail chest and Intercostal drain placement. This block is also given for chronic pain management in cases of post-herpetic neuralgia [42–49].

Complications Pneumothorax is a known complication.

Ultrasound technique Patient decubitus: lateral, sitting or prone. A high-frequency linear array transducer is used. The ribs are identified by their curved hyperechogenic surface outline and the acoustic shadow underneath them in a parasagittal view (Between adjacent ribs, the intercostal muscles, and pleura is identified (hyperechoic line in gliding motion during respiration). Initial scanning is performed in the transverse plane of the rib to identify the level. The level of the block is marked by counting the ribs from above downwards starting from second rib or in the opposite direction starting from the 12th rib [40, 41]. Another landmark used is T7 at the level of the tip of scapula [41]. The ideal point to block the nerve is at the angle of the rib (6–7 cm lateral to the spinous process) before the nerves branches out [42, 43]. The neurovascular bundle lies between the internal intercostal and the innermost intercostal muscles.

In plane or out of plane approach can be used. It is very important to identify the plane by hydrodissection at every level to prevent damage to the pleura [44, 45] or the vascular bundle lying in close proximity to the nerve. It is prudent to check for pneumothorax by seeing the gliding movement of the pleura and the comet tail appearance underneath (they both disappear in the case of pnemothorax [45]. Once the correct plane is reached 3–5 mL of local anaesthetic solution should be injected after careful aspiration. The needle is introduced usually from the superior border of the rib below.

4.3.4 Interpleural Block

LA is injected between the two layers of pleura. It is effective for thoracic and upper abdominal surgeries. Some centres regularly practice this block, while others refrain from it citing the reported 2% incidence of pneumothorax among other complications such as pleural infection and adhesion [50, 51]. Landmark-based technique using a saline infusion has been practiced widely [52]. The use of ultrasound is expected to bring down the complication rate.

Ultrasound Technique Patient can be in sitting, lateral, semi-prone or prone position. A high-frequency linear UST is held transversely to image the pleura at fifth–sixth intercostal space in the posterior axillary line. The two layers of pleura may be difficult to identify. The needle is inserted in a plane to breach the internal intercostal membrane, directly beneath which lies the pleura, which can be seen as a shiny white line. The needle then is very slowly inserted further to breach the parietal pleura. A saline infusion technique can be used for additional safety to find out the interpleural space. A saline drip is attached to the block needle and made air free in the beginning. Interpleural space being a negative pressure space, the saline starts flowing freely once the needle enters the parietal pleura. Alternatively, a loss of resistance (LOR) syringe can also be used [53, 54]. A catheter can be placed in situ for continuous analgesia.

Indications Interpleural block has been shown to provide safe, high-quality analgesia after cholecystectomy, thoracotomy, renal and breast surgery, and invasive radiological procedures of the renal and hepatobiliary systems. It has been used successfully in the treatment of pain from multiple rib fractures, herpes zoster, complex regional pain syndromes, thoracic and abdominal cancer and pancreatitis [53–55].

Complications Pneumothorax, pleural infection and adhesion are known complications.

4.4 Blocks in the Back

4.4.1 Erector Spinae Plain (ESP) Block

Anatomy

Erector spinae is a group of muscles comprising iliocostalis, longissimus and spinalis which runs from the base of the skull to the median crest of the sacrum (Figs. 4.21 and 4.22). Erector spinae plane (ESP) block is a novel interfascial paraspinal plane block first described by Forero et al. in 2016 [56], in which LA is deposited over the transverse process, which is about 3 cm lateral to the spinous process, deep to the three columns of ES muscle. LA diffuses across interfascial planes and reaches paravertebral space via a costotransverse groove. Block action is

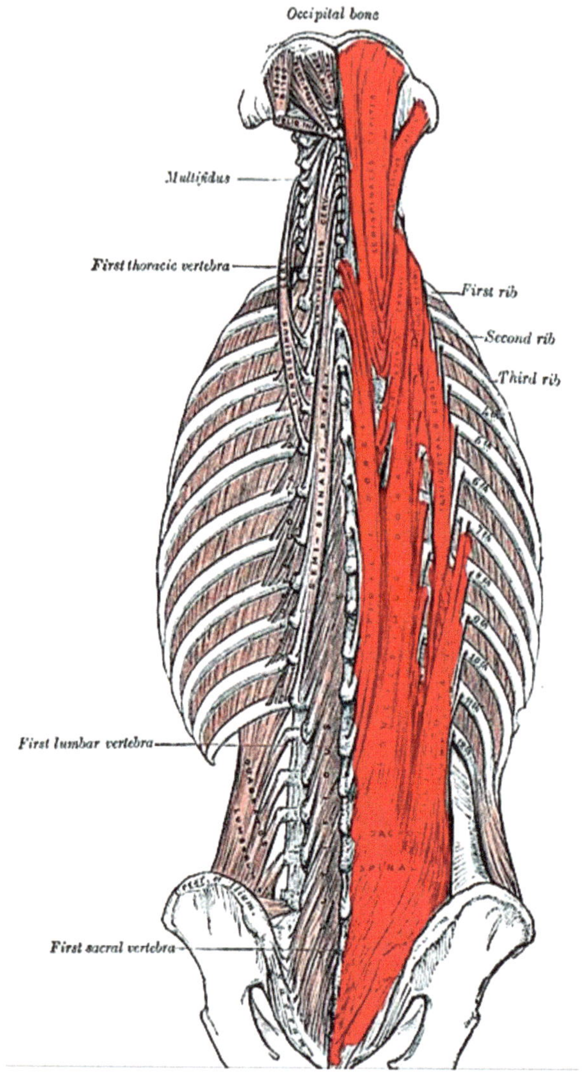

Fig. 4.21 Red highlighted structures indicate the three columns of the erector spinae muscles. Medial to lateral: spinalis, longissimus, iliocostalis

predominantly via dorsal rami and also at times via ventral rami (especially in the thoracic region) [56, 57].

A single shot ESP provides the benefit of a multilevel thoracic paravertebral block (TPVB) without the risks of TPVB. Since introduction, it has become rapidly popular as a choice of technique for regional anaesthesia as well as interventional pain management.

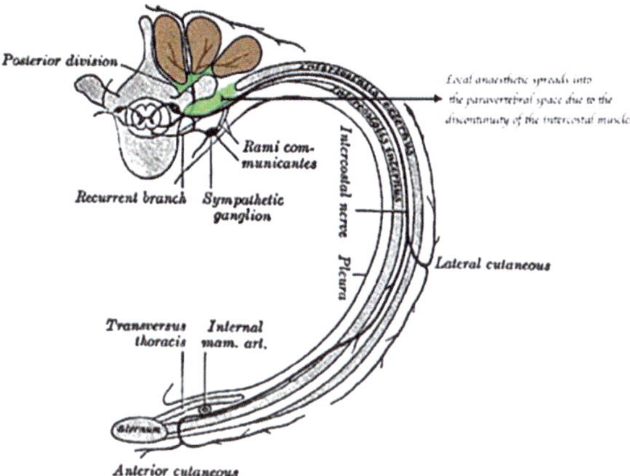

Fig. 4.22 Anatomy relation of ESP muscle, transverse process, costotransverse groove, dorsal and ventral rami with its branches

While the endpoint for injection in the thoracic and lumbar level is the lateral edge of the transverse process, in the sacral level, the endpoint is the intermediate crest of the sacrum.

Patient Position Prone, sitting or lateral decubitus position.

Ultrasound Technique
A high-frequency linear or curvilinear (in obese) probe is placed in the parasagittal or transverse plane. Both in plane and out of plane techniques can be used. Spinous process is first identified in the transverse imaging and then moving about 3 cm laterally the transverse process can be imaged. LA is deposited at the edge of the transverse process (seen as a hyperechoic square pattern on USG). Hydrodissection helps in preventing inadvertent intramuscular injection in ES muscle. Block can be performed at any level starting from cervical region to sacral level depending on the indications. Multilevel injections or continuous ESP catheter either unilateral or bilateral can be used in selected cases for better quality of analgesia. Block action is checked after block completion [58] (Figs. 4.23, 4.24 and 4.25).

Drugs and dosages Single injection at T4/T5 or at T8/T9 using a volume of 0.3 mg/kg produces adequate analgesia in isolated hemithorax and hemiabdomen respectively.

Usual concentration is 0.2–0.375% ropivacaine or 0.125–0.25% bupivacaine or levobupivacaine with or without 4 mg dexamethasone as adjuvant can be employed. All interfascial plane blocks work well when combined with multimodal analgesia.

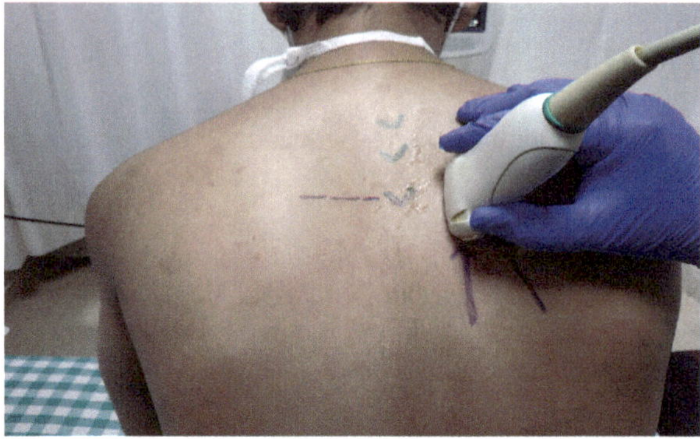

Fig. 4.23 Probe position parasagittal in plane technique for Erector Spinae Plane Block

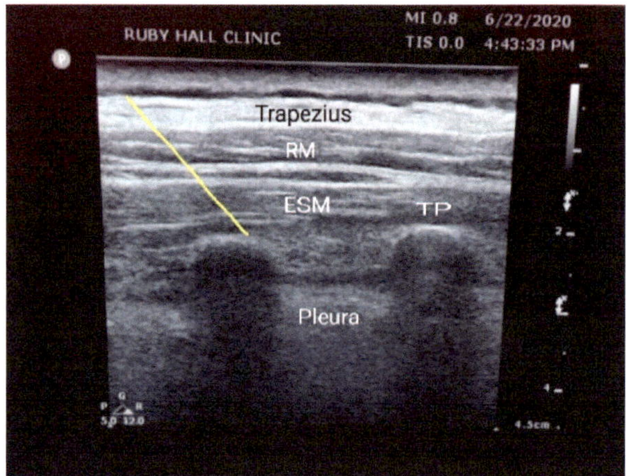

Fig. 4.24 Ultrasound Image of Erector Spinae Plane Block at the thoracic level. LA deposited at the edge of transverse process beneath erector spinae muscle

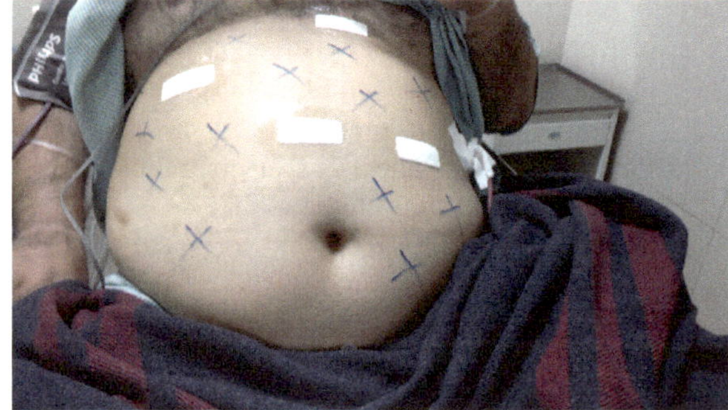

Fig. 4.25 Assessment of sensory level (T6-L1) with ice after performing bilateral ESPB block at T8 level in a case of laparoscopic sleeve gastrectomy

Indications

1. Thoracic: VATS and Open thoracic surgeries, fracture ribs, breast surgeries, open cardiac surgeries [59–63] (Fig. 4.26).
2. Abdominal: Laparoscopic cholecystectomy, gastric bypass [64], PCNL, renal transplant, caesarean section, midline laparotomies.

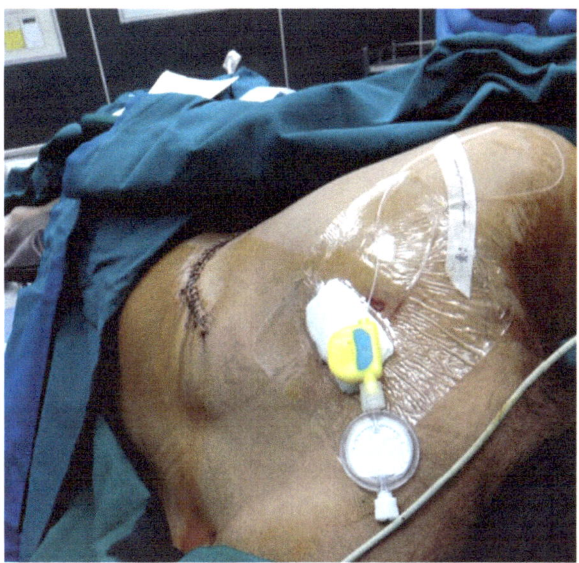

Fig. 4.26 Erector spinae continuous catheter in a case of breast surgery with latissimus dorsi flap

3. Novel indications: ASIS bone graft, hip and femur surgery (e.g. at L4 level), refractory headache, chronic shoulder pain, chronic thoracic neuropathic pain, spine surgery as rescue block for breakthrough post-surgical pain [65–68].
4. Thoracic ESP block has been used for management of back pain due to a wide variety of causes, such as radiculopathy and vertebral fracture.
5. Sacral erector spinae block has been used for analgesia for perineal surgeries and for radicular pain management.

Complications They are rare as per case reports. Minimal hypotension or lower limb weakness due to the spread of LA in epidural space has been reported [66].

Blockmate Pearls

- ESP is a versatile block that can be used from the cervical to the sacral level.
- ESP for breast surgery has the advantage of covering all the dermatomes in a single injection compared with thoracic paravertebral, where multiple injections have to be made.
- ESP retains all the benefits of TPVB while being free from the complications that come with TPVB.

4.4.2 Thoracolumbar Interfascial Plane (TLIP) Block

The TLIP block is another paraspinal fascial plane block which was described earlier to ESPB and is similar to ESPB albeit with different injection endpoint and technique.

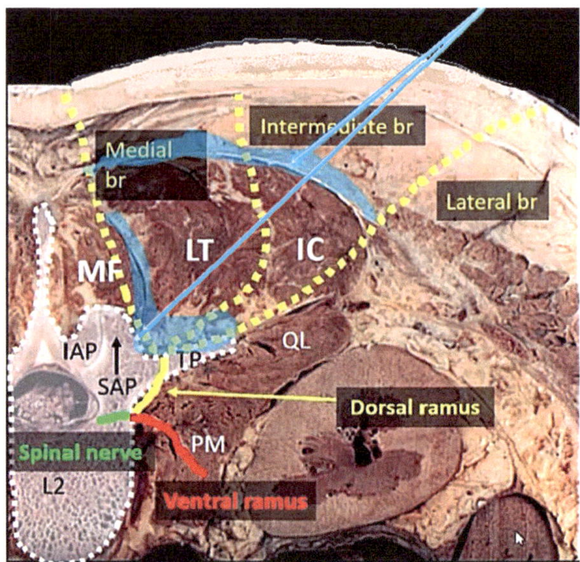

Fig. 4.27 TLIP anatomy and deposition of LA: Arrows represent needle trajectory, blue coloured area spread of LA, *PM* psoas major, *QL* quadratus lumborum, *IC* iliocostalis, *LT* longissimus thoracis, *MF* multifidus muscle, *L2* second lumbar vertebra, *SAP* superior articular process, *IAP* inferior articular process, *TP* transverse process

Anatomy TLIP is modification of ESPB block, first described by Hand and colleagues in 2015 [69]. ESP muscle has the following three muscle groups from medial to lateral namely Multifidus, longissimus thoracis and Iliocostalis in the lumbar area. Dorsal rami divides into medial, lateral and intermediate branches at the base of multifidus and longissimus thoracis muscle. As the injection endpoint suggests, TLIP works on the dorsal rami, not the ventral (Fig. 4.27).

Indications Post-operative analgesia for all lumbar spine surgeries, spinal cord stimulator implant insertion procedures.

USG Procedure Curvilinear probe is commonly used. Block is usually performed bilaterally. Patient is given a prone position. Transverse paramedian scan on either side of the spinous process in the lumbar area to identify erector spinae muscle morphology is the first step. LA (15–20 mL) is deposited between the plane between multifidus and longissimus thoracis closer to the superior articular process. LA spreads proximally to block all branches of dorsal rami [69, 70]. Additional second injection (5 mL) in the skin and subcutaneous tissue over ESP muscle ensures better coverage of subcutaneous nerve branches. The drug concentration used for this block is 0.2% ropivacaine or 0.125% bupivacaine or levobupivacaine (Fig. 4.28).

Blockmate Pearls

- TLIP is indicated for spine surgery, low back pain, post spine surgery pain syndrome, etc.
- Although its use is limited, the analgesia provided by TLIP in its described area is dense.
- Due to the anatomical structure of the lumbar vertebrae, the superior articular process is imaged in the same plane as the spinous process (spine), making the imaging easier. The transverse process lies a little cephalad to the spine.

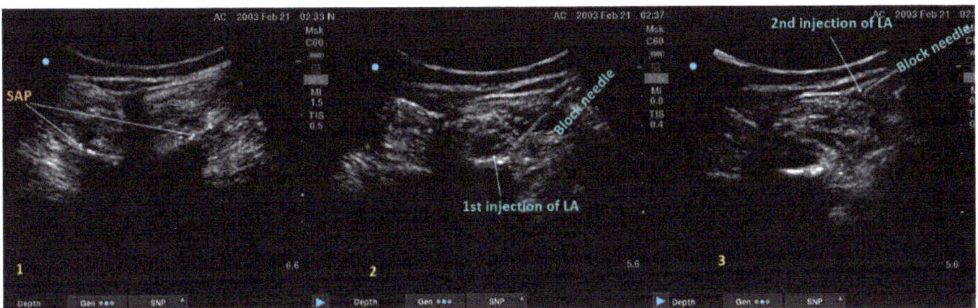

Fig. 4.28 Ultrasound-guided TLIP block: (1) Sonoanatomy showing the hypoechoic shadow of the Lumbar spine and hyperechoic reflection of the superior articular process (SAP). (2) Block needle is seen entering in plane and striking the SAP. First LA injection is given above the SAP. (3) The block needle is withdrawn and a second injection of LA is put between the thoracolumbar fascia and the iliocostalis muscle

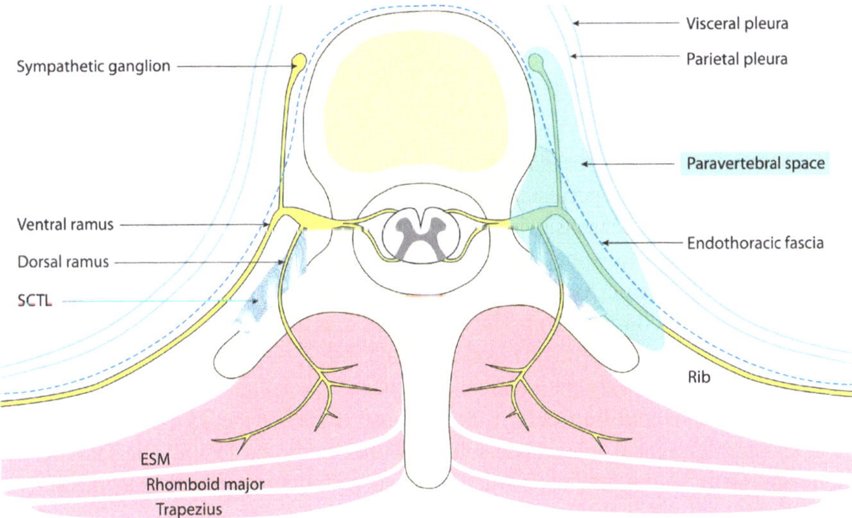

Fig. 4.29 Anatomy of thoracic paravertebral space: *SCTL* superior costotransverse ligament. Pawa A, Wojcikiewicz T, Barron A. et al. Paravertebral Blocks: Anatomical, Practical, and Future Concepts. Curr Anesthesiol Rep. 2019;9:263–270. https://doi.org/10.1007/s40140-019-00328-x

4.4.3 Thoracic Paravertebral Block (TPVB)

Anatomy First described by Sellheim in 1905, the thoracic paravertebral block (TPVB) is an ipsilateral somatosensory and sympathetic nerve block at multiple different levels [71–75]. The thoracic paravertebral space (TPVS) is a wedge-shaped space bordering the vertebral bodies extending from T1-T12, located on either side of the vertebral column (Figs. 4.29 and 4.30). The parietal pleura forms the anterolateral boundary. The base is formed by the vertebral body, intervertebral disc and the intervertebral foramen with its contents. The transverse process and the superior costotransverse ligament form the posterior boundary. Lying in between the parietal pleura anteriorly and the superior costotransverse ligament posteriorly is the endo-

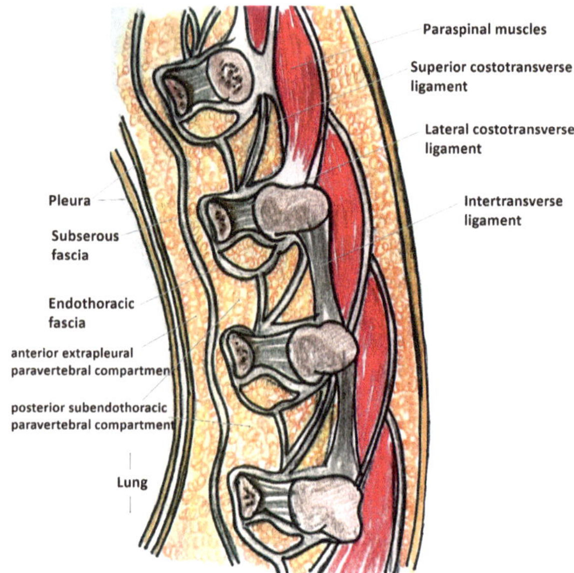

Fig. 4.30 Sagittal section through the paravertebral space

thoracic fascia, which is the deep fascia of the thorax. Medially, the endothoracic fascia is attached to the periosteum of the vertebral body. A layer of loose areolar connective tissue, the subserous fascia, lies between the parietal pleura and the endothoracic fascia. Therefore, there are two potential fascial compartments in the TPVS: the anterior extrapleural paravertebral compartment and the posterior subendothoracic paravertebral compartment. The TPVS contains adipose tissue within which lie the intercostal (spinal) nerve, the dorsal ramus, intercostal vessels, and rami communicantes and anteriorly the sympathetic chain. The spinal nerves are segmented into small bundles and lie freely in the adipose tissue of the TPVS, which makes them accessible to local anaesthetic solutions injected in the TPVS. The TPVS communicates with the epidural space medially and with the intercostal space laterally.

Indications

1. Analgesia: Rib fractures, herpetic neuralgia, cancer pain, complex regional pain syndrome.
2. Surgical anaesthesia and post-operative analgesia for breast [76, 77], thoracic [74] and abdominal surgeries (e.g. cholecystectomy, appendicectomy, hernia repair, etc.)

Complications

1. Pneumothorax (Incidence 0.5%)
2. Epidural spread of LA causing hypotension
3. Reversible side effects like Horner's syndrome if the block is performed at T1/T2 level
4. Local anaesthetic systemic toxicity (LAST)

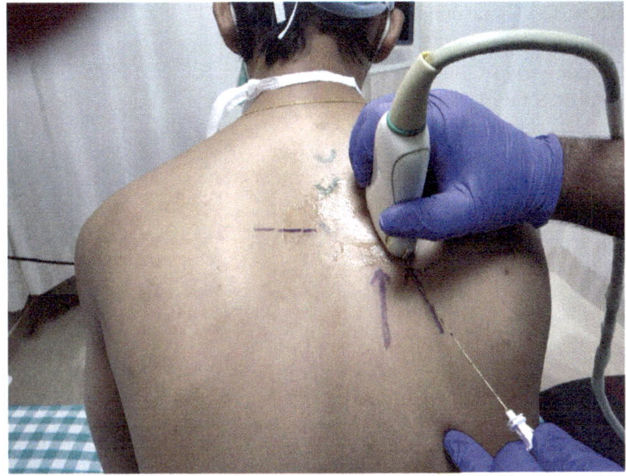

Fig. 4.31 Probe position parasagittal oblique in plane technique for TPVB

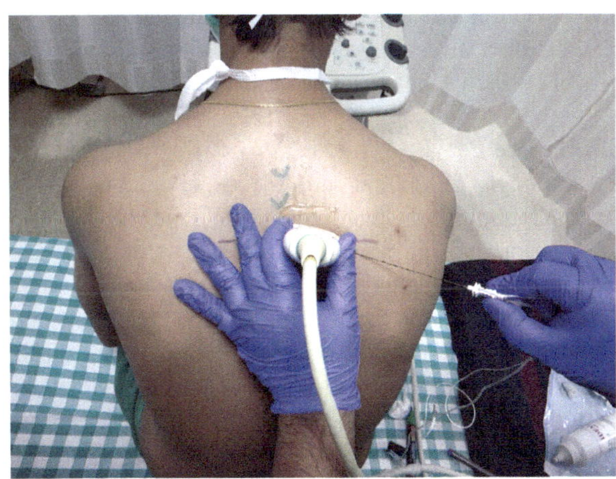

Fig. 4.32 Probe position transverse in plane technique for TPVB

USG Technique High-frequency linear or curvilinear probe is used with the patient in a sitting position (with curved back) or lateral (fetal) position.

A common technique is parasagittal oblique scan using either in plane or out of plane method (Fig. 4.31). Another technique popularized by Dr. Manoj Karmakar et al. is a transverse scan using in plane technique (Fig. 4.32). Both the techniques are highly demanding and should be done only under expert supervision until sufficient experience is obtained.

Sonoanatomy Landmark Identification of transverse process, ribs, pleura, lung, wedge-shaped paravertebral space and costotransverse ligament [78] (Fig. 4.33). Anterior displacement of parietal pleura with correct deposition of LA in paravertebral space is the telltale sign of a proper block [76, 77, 79].

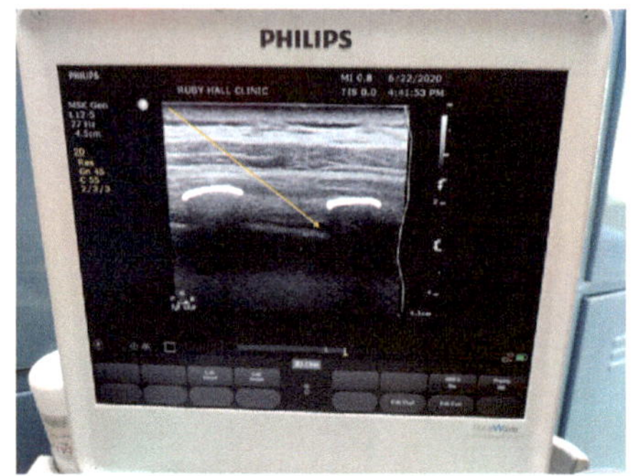

Fig. 4.33 Ultrasound Image of parasagittal oblique view of thoracic paravertebral block (TPVB) showing transverse process (white line), direction on needle (yellow line) within PVB space and the underlying pleura

Dose

1. Surgical Anaesthesia: 0.375–0.5% Ropivacaine or Bupivacaine or Levobupivacaine in the dose of 3–5 mL at each level. Multilevel injections with or without a catheter are preferred methods.
2. Post-operative analgesia: 0.3 mL/kg or 15–20 mL of 0.2% ropivacaine or 0.125–0.25% bupivacaine or levobupivacaine with or without adjuvants.

Blockmate Pearls

- Although TPVB can provide excellent analgesia for thoracic surgeries, the manipulation of chest wall muscles such as pectoralis major, minor, serratus anterior and latissimus dorsi evoke pain as these muscles are innervated by branches of brachial plexus which have a much higher (C5-T1) origin compared to the level of the paravertebral block (T3-T6).
- Multilevel TPVB is required for surgical anaesthesia for thoracic surgery. ESPB on the other hand covers multiple dermatomal levels in a single injection. Hence following advent of the ESPB, TPVB has fallen out of favour. ESPB is a safer and easier alternative.
- Higher volume of LA injected in TPVB can cause hypotension due to epidural spread.
- Higher volume of LA injected in TPVB on one side can theoretically block the other side as the two spaces are connected by prevertebral space.

References

1. Hebbard P, Fujiwara Y, Shibata Y, Royse C. Ultrasound-guided TAM plane (TAP) block. Anaesth Intensive Care. 2007;35:616–7.
2. Rozen WM, Tran TM, Ashton MW, Barrington MJ, Ivanusic JJ, Taylor GI. Refining the course of the thoracolumbar nerves: a new understanding of the innervation of the anterior abdominal wall. Clin Anat. 2008;21:325–33.
3. Rafi A. Abdominal field block: a new approach via the lumbar triangle. Anaesthesia. 2001;56:24–6.

4. McDonnell JG, O'Donnell B, Curley G, Heffernan A, Power C, Laffey JG. The analgesic efficacy of TAM plane block after abdominal surgery: a prospective randomized controlled trial. Anesth Analg. 2007;104:193–7.
5. Carney J, Finnerty O, Rauf J, Bergin D, Laffey JG, Mc Donnell JG. Studies on the spread of LA solution in TAM plane blocks. Anaesthesia. 2011;66:1023–30.
6. Abdallah FW, Chan VW, Brull R. TAM plane block: the effects of surgery, dosing, technique, and timing on analgesic outcomes. A systematic review. Reg Anesth Pain Med. 2012;37:193–209.
7. Abdallah FW, Laffey JG, Halpern SH, Brull R. Duration of analgesic effectiveness after the posterior and lateral TAM plane block techniques for transverse lower abdominal incisions: a meta-analysis. Br J Anaesth. 2013;111:721–35.
8. Hebbard PD, Barrington MJ, Vasey C. Ultrasound-guided continuous oblique subcostal TAM plane blockade: description of anatomy and clinical technique. Reg Anesth Pain Med. 2010;35:436–41.
9. Børglum J, Maschmann C, Belhage B, Jensen K. Ultrasound-guided bilateral dual TAM plane block: a new four-point approach. Acta Anaesthesiol Scand. 2011;55:658–63.
10. Børglum J, Jensen K, Christensen AF, Hoegberg LC, Johansen SS, Lönnqvist PA, et al. Distribution patterns, dermatomal anaesthesia and ropivacaine serum concentrations after bilateral dual TAM plane block. Reg Anesth Pain Med. 2012;37:294–301.
11. Niraj G, Kelkar A, Hart E, Horst C, Malik D, Yeow C, et al. Comparison of analgesic efficacy of four-quadrant TAM plane (TAP) block and continuous posterior TAP analgesia with epidural analgesia in patients undergoing laparoscopic colorectal surgery: an open-label, randomised, non-inferiority trial. Anaesthesia. 2014;69:348–53.
12. Toshniwal G, Soskin V. Ultrasound guided transversus abdominis plane block in obese patients. Indian J Anaesth. 2012;56:104–5.
13. Sandeman DJ, Dilley AV. Ultrasound-guided rectus sheath block and catheter placement. ANZ J Surg. 2008;78:621–3
14. Cornish P, Deacon A. Rectus sheath catheters for continuous analgesia after upper abdominal surgery. ANZ J Surg. 2007;77:84.
15. Blanco R. Optimal point of injection: the quadratus lumborum type I and II blocks. http://www.respond2articles.com/ANA/forums/post/1550.aspx.
16. Sauter AR, Ullensvang K, Niemi G, Lorentzen HT, Bendtsen TF, Børglum J, et al. The Shamrock lumbar plexus block: a dose-finding study. Eur J Anaesthesiol. 2015;32:764–70.
17. Kadam VR. Ultrasound-guided quadratus lumborum block as a postoperative analgesic technique for laparotomy. J Anaesthesiol Clin Pharmacol. 2013;29:550–2.
18. Visoiu M, Yakovleva N. Continuous postoperative analgesia via quadratus lumborum block—an alternative to TAM plane block. Paediatr Anaesth. 2013;23:959–61.
19. Chakraborty A, Goswami J, Patro V. Ultrasound-guided continuous quadratus lumborum block for postoperative analgesia in a pediatric patient. A A Case Rep. 2015;4:34–6.
20. Ecoffey C. Regional anaesthesia in children. In: Raj PP, editor. Textbook of regional anaesthesia. Philadelphia, PA: Churchill Livingstone; 2002. p. 379–93.
21. Kopacz DL, Thompson GE. Celiac and hypogastric plexus, intercostal, interpleural and peripheral neural blockade of the thorax and abdomen. In: Cousins MJ, Bridenbaugh PO, editors. Neural blockade in clinical anaesthesia and management of pain. Philadelphia, PA: Lippincott; 1998. p. 451–85.
22. Reynolds L, Kedlaya D. Ilioinguinal-iliohypogastric and genitofemoral nerve blocks. In: Waldman SD, editor. Interventional pain management. Philadelphia: WB Saunders; 2001. p. 508–11.
23. Waldman SD. Ilioinguinal and iliohypogastric nerve block. In: Waldman SD, editor. Atlas of interventional pain management. Philadelphia: Saunders; 2004. p. 294–301.
24. Willschke H, Marhofer P, Bosenberg A, et al. Ultrasonography for ilioinguinal/iliohypogastric nerve blocks in children. Br J Anaesth. 2005;95:226–30.

25. Eichenberger U, Greher M, Kirchmair L, et al. Ultrasound-guided blocks of the ilioinguinal and iliohypogastric nerve: accuracy of a selective new technique confirmed by anatomical dissection. Br J Anaesth. 2006;97:238–43.
26. Aveline C, Le Hetet H, Le Roux A. Comparison between ultrasound-guided TAM plane and conventional ilioinguinal/iliohypogastric nerve blocks for day-case open inguinal hernia repair. Br J Anaesth. 2011;106:380–6.
27. Gofeld M, Christakis M. Sonographically guided ilioinguinal nerve block. J Ultrasound Med. 2006;25:1571–5.
28. Lee S, Tan JSK. Ultrasonography-guided ilioinguinal-iliohypogastric nerve block for inguinal herniotomies in ex-premature Neonates. Singapore Med J. 2013;54:218–20.
29. Shanthanna H. Successful treatment of genitofemoral neuralgia using ultrasound guided injection: a case report and short review of literature. Case Rep Anesthesiol. 2014;2014:371703.
30. Wipfli M, Birkhäuser F, Luyet C. Ultrasound guided spermatic cord block for scrotal surgery. Br J Anaesth. 2011;106:255–9.
31. Birkhäuser FD, Wipfli M, Eichenberger U, Luyet C, Greif R, Thalmann GN. Vasectomy reversal with ultrasonography-guided spermatic cord block. BJU Int. 2012;110:1796–800.
32. Porzionato A, Macchi V, Stecco C, Loukas M, Tubbs RS, De Caro R. Surgical anatomy of the pectoral nerves and the pectoral musculature. Clin Anat. 2012;25:559–75.
33. Macéa JR, Fregnani JHTG. Anatomy of the thoracic wall, axilla and breast. Int J Morphol. 2006;24:691–704.
34. Blanco R. The 'pecs block': a novel technique for providing analgesia after breast surgery. Anaesthesia. 2011;66:847–8.
35. Blanco R, Fajardo M, Parras Maldonado T. Ultrasound description of Pecs II (modified Pecs I): a novel approach to breast surgery. Rev Esp Anestesiol Reanim. 2012;59:470–5.
36. Pérez MF, Miguel JG, de la Torre PA. A new approach to pectoralis block. Anaesthesia. 2013;68:430.
37. Blanco R, Parras T, McDonnell JG, Prats-Galino A. Serratus plane block: a novel ultrasound-guided thoracic wall nerve block. Anaesthesia. 2013;68:1107–13.
38. Tighe SQ, Karmakar MK. Serratus plane block: do we need to learn another technique for thoracic wall blockade? Anaesthesia. 2013;68:1103–6.
39. Madabushi R, Tewari S, Gautam SK, et al. Serratus anterior plane block: a new analgesic technique for post-thoracotomy pain. Pain Physician. 2015;18:E421–4.
40. Moore DC. Anatomy of the intercostal nerve: its importance during thoracic surgery. Am J Surg. 1982;144:371–3.
41. Bhatia A, Gofeld M, Ganapathy S, Hanlon J, Johnson M. Comparison of anatomic landmarks and ultrasound guidance for intercostal nerve injections in cadavers. Reg Anesth Pain Med. 2013;38:503–7.
42. Peng PWHBS, Narouze S. Ultrasound-guided interventional procedures in pain medicine: a review of anatomy, sonoanatomy, and procedures: Part I: Nonaxial structures. Reg Anesth Pain Med. 2009;34:458–74.
43. Moore DC, Bridenbaugh LD. Intercostal nerve block: indications, technique and complications. Anesth Analg. 1962;41:1–10.
44. Shanti CM, Carlin AM, Tyburski JG. Incidence of pneumothorax from intercostal nerve block for analgesia in rib fractures. J Trauma. 2001;51:536–9.
45. Reissig A, Kroegel C. Accuracy of transthoracic sonography in excluding post-interventional pneumothorax and hydropneumothorax: comparison to chest radiography. Eur J Radiol. 2005;53:463–70.
46. Curatolo M, Eichenberger U. Ultrasound-guided blocks for the treatment of chronic pain. Techniques Reg Anaesth Pain Manag. 2007;11:95–102.
47. Byas-Smith MG, Gulati A. Ultrasound-guided intercostal nerve cryoablation. Anesth Analg. 2006;103:1033–5.
48. Shankar H, Eastwood D. Retrospective comparison of ultrasound and fluoroscopic image guidance for intercostal steroid injections. Pain Pract. 2010;10:312–7.

49. Ozkan D, Akkaya T, Karakoyunlu N, Arik E, Ergil J, Koc Z, et al. Effect of ultrasound-guided intercostal nerve block on postoperative pain after percutaneous nephrolithotomy: prospective randomized controlled study. Anaesthesist. 2013;62:988–94.
50. Morris CJ, Bunsell R. Intrapleural blocks for chest wall surgery. Anaesthesia. 2014;69(1):85–6.
51. Strømskag KE, Minor BG, Steen PA. Side effects and complications related to interpleural analgesia: an update. Acta Anaesthesiol Scand. 1990;34:473–7.
52. Scott PV. Interpleural regional analgesia: detection of the interpleural space by saline infusion. Br J Anaesth. 1991;66:131–3.
53. Dravid RM, Paul RE. Interpleural block – part 1. Anaesthesia. 2007;62:1039–49.
54. Dravid RM, Paul RE. Interpleural block – part 2. Anaesthesia. 2007;62:1143–53.
55. Sadana M, Mayall M. Interpleural blocks and clotting abnormalities: a case report. Anaesthesia. 2008;63:553.
56. Forero M, Adhikary SD, Lopez H, Tsui C, Chin KJ. The erector spinae plane block: a novel analgesic technique in thoracic neuropathic pain. Reg Anesth Pain Med. 2016;41(5):621–7.
57. Schwartzmann A, Peng P, Maciel MA, et al. Mechanism of the erector spinae plane block: insights from a magnetic resonance imaging study. Can J Anaesth. 2018;65:1165–6.
58. Chin KJ, McDonnell JG, Carvalho B, Sharkey A, Pawa A, Gadsden J. Essentials of our current understanding: abdominal wall blocks. Reg Anesth Pain Med. 2017;42:133–83.
59. Adhikary SD, Liu WM, Fuller E, Cruz-Eng H, Chin KJ. The effect of erector spinae plane block on respiratory and analgesic outcomes in multiple rib fractures: a retrospective cohort study. Anaesthesia. 2019;74(5):585–93.
60. Ciftci B, Ekinci M, Cem Celik E, Cem Tukac I, Bayrak Y, Oktay Atalay Y. Efficacy of an ultrasound-guided erector spinae plane block for postoperative analgesia management after video-assisted thoracic surgery: a prospective randomized study. J Cardiothorac Vasc Anesth. 2019. pii:S1053-0770(19)30407-0.
61. Nath S, Bhoi D, Mohan VK, Talawar P. USG-guided continuous erector spinae block as a primary mode of perioperative analgesia in open posterolateral thoracotomy: a report of two cases. Saudi J Anaesth. 2018;12(3):471–4.
62. Gurkan Y, Aksu C, Kus ¨ A, Yorukoglu UH, Kılıc CT. Ultrasound guided erector spinae plane block reduces postoperative, opioid consumption following breast surgery: a randomized controlled study. J Clin Anesth. 2018;50:65–8.
63. Krishna SN, Chauhan S, Bhoi D, et al. Bilateral erector spinae plane block for acute post-surgical pain in adult cardiac surgical patients: a randomized controlled trial. J Cardiothorac Vasc Anesth. 2019;33(2):368–75.
64. Chin KJ, Malhas L, Perlas A. The erector spinae plane block provides visceral abdominal analgesia in bariatric surgery a report of 3 cases. Reg Anesth Pain Med. 2017;42(3):372–6.
65. Tulgar S, Kose HC, Selvi O, et al. Comparison of ultrasound-guided lumbar erector spinae plane block and transmuscular quadratus lumborum block for postoperative analgesia in hip and proximal femur surgery: a prospective randomized feasibility study. Anesth Essays Res. 2018;12(4):825–31.
66. Selvi O, Tulgar S. Ultrasound guided erector spinae plane block as a cause of unintended motor block. Rev Esp Anestesiol Reanim. 2018;65(10):589–92.
67. Ueshima H, Inagaki M, Toyone T, Otake H. Efficacy of the erector spinae plane block for lumbar spinal surgery: a retrospective study. Asian Spine J. 2019;13(2):254–7.
68. Ueshima H, Otake H. Successful cases of bilateral erector spinae plane block for treatment of tension headache. J Clin Anesth. 2019;54:153.
69. Hand W, Taylor J. TLIP block. Can J Anesth. 2015;62:1196–200.
70. Aniskalioglu A, Yayik AM. USG guided lateral TLIP. J Clin Anesth. 2017;40:62. https://doi.org/10.1016/j.clinane.2017.04.015.
71. Conacher ID. Resin injection of thoracic paravertebral spaces. Br J Anaesth. 1988;61(6):657–61.
72. Naja Z, Lonnqvist PA. Somatic paravertebral nerve blockade. Incidence of failed block and complications. Anaesthesia. 2001;56(12):1184–8.

73. Pace MM, Sharma B, Anderson-Dam J, Fleischmann K, Warren L, Stefanovich P. Ultrasound-guided thoracic paravertebral blockade: a retrospective study of the incidence of complications. Anesth Analg. 2016;122(4):1186–91.
74. Uskova A, LaColla L, Albani F, Auroux AS, Chelly JE. Comparison of ultrasound-assisted and classic approaches to continuous paravertebral block for video-assisted thoracoscopic surgery: a prospective randomized trial. Int J Anesthesiol Res. 2015;3(1):9–16.
75. Cowie B, McGlade D, Ivanusic J, Barrington MJ. Ultrasound-guided thoracic paravertebral blockade: a cadaveric study. Anesth Analg. 2010;110(6):1735–9.
76. O Riain SC, Donnell BO, Cuffe T, Harmon DC, Fraher JP, Shorten G. Thoracic paravertebral block using real-time ultrasound guidance. Anesth Analg. 2010;110(1):248–51.
77. Hara K, Sakura S, Nomura T, Saito Y. Ultrasound guided thoracic paravertebral block in breast surgery. Anaesthesia. 2009;64(2):223–5.
78. Pusch F, Wildling E, Klimscha W, Weinstabl C. Sonographic measurement of needle insertion depth in paravertebral blocks in women. Br J Anaesth. 2000;85(6):841–3.
79. Karmakar M. Musculoskeletal ultrasound for regional anaesthesia and pain medicine. 2nd ed; 2016. p. 345–70.

Central Neuraxial Blockade

5

Swati Parmar and Balakrishnan Ashokka

List of Abbreviations

ASA	Anterior Spinal Artery
CSE	Combined spinal epidural
CSF	Cerebrospinal fluid
LA	Local anaesthetics
LAST	Local Anaesthetic Systemic Toxicity
LDNP	Large dural needle puncture
PDPH	Post Dural Puncture Headache
PSA	Posterior Spinal Artery
SAB	Subarachnoid block
SCL	Sacrococcygeal ligament
TP	Transverse process
USG	Ultrasonongrahy

5.1 Anatomy

Neuraxial Space The spinal column (Fig. 5.1)extends from the base of the skull up to the lower part of the pelvis.

Bone The spinal column has 33 vertebrae. For a central neuraxial block, the anatomy of a typical lumbar vertebra is relevant. Each vertebra has two main components i.e. Body and Posterior vertebral arch. The vertebral arch further contains pedicle, lamina, superior and inferior articulating surfaces as described in Fig. 5.2. The projecting processes in vertebrae are two transverse processes laterally, one

S. Parmar (✉) · B. Ashokka
Department of Anaesthesia, National University Hospital, Singapore, Singapore

A. Chakraborty (ed.), *Blockmate*, https://doi.org/10.1007/978-981-15-9202-7_5

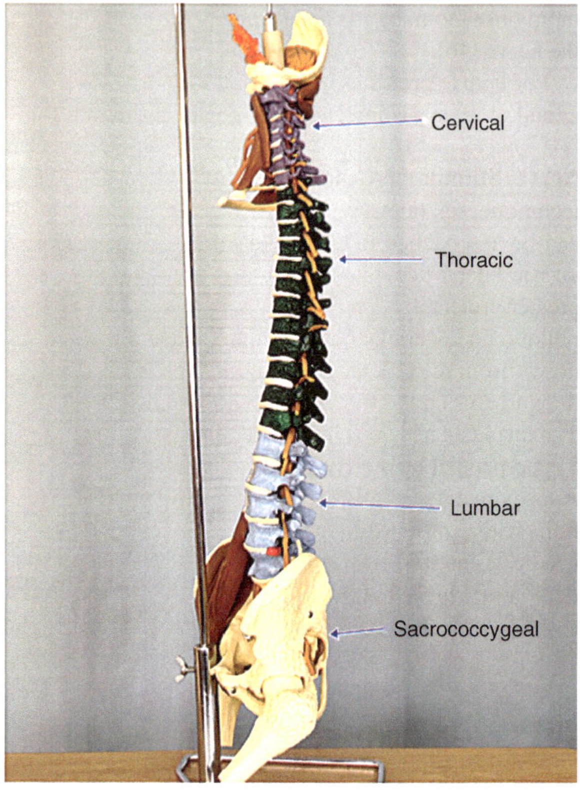

Fig. 5.1 Spinal segments extending from base of the skull to pelvis

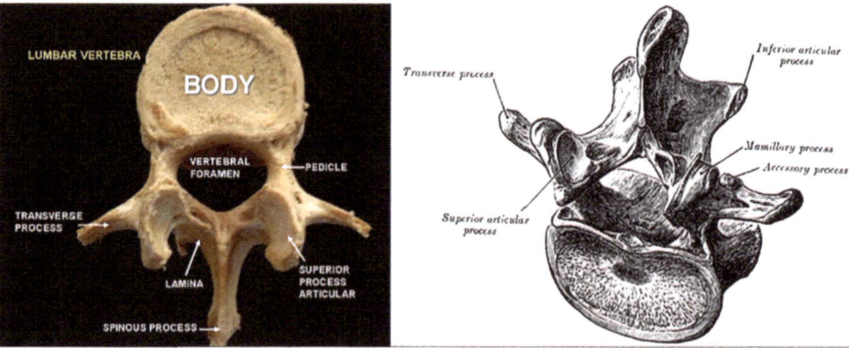

Fig. 5.2 Typical lumbar vertebrae: Image source: Wikimedia commons. Digitally modified and rendered by Dr. Arunangshu Chakraborty

spinous process posteriorly both arising from the lamina/vertebral body, two superior articulating and two inferior articulating processes.

The lumbar vertebral column is convex forward with each vertebra having a large kidney-shaped body, a non-bifid spinous process and an arch posteriorly that is formed by thick pedicles, short and thick transverse process and triangular vertebral foramina. The vertebral arch encroaches the body leaving a gap in the centre for the

Table 5.1 Ligaments of the spinal column

Ligaments	Extent	Remarks
Supraspinous	Tip of C7 spine to the sacrum	Thick band which thins out at lumbar level. First to encounter while performing a midline neuraxial approach.
Interspinous	Anteriorly from ligamentum flavum to posteriorly supraspinous ligaments.	Second lig. to encounter while performing midline neuraxial.
Ligamentum flavum	Connects lamina of adjacent vertebrae.	Dense elastic lig. and responsible for LOR technique of epidural as it is encountered. Thickness is usually 3–5 mm.
The posterior longitudinal	Lies posterior to the vertebra and intervertebral discs.	
The anterior longitudinal	Anterior to body/intervertebral discs and extends from C2 to sacrum	

spinal cord to pass through it. The contents of the spinal canal are spinal cord, spinal nerves and vessels.

5.1.1 Intervertebral Discs and Ligaments

Each vertebra is attached to its adjacent vertebra with the help of facet joints and distinguishes patterns of ligaments which equally take part in stability, movements and weight transmission.

The cushion of the neuraxial column, the *intervertebral discs* has a central component of disc which is gelatinous, soft, avascular elastic tissue, embryonic in origin, *nucleosus pulposus* (Fig. 5.2). Surrounding this is the layer of concentric rings of fibrocartilage, *annular ligaments*.

There are few important ligaments relevant (Table 5.1) to the anatomy of it while performing Spinal/Epidural anaesthesia.

The ligamentum nuchae is the ligamentum flavum above T7 attaches to the occipital external protuberance.

Joints The superior and inferior articular processes arising from the junction of the lamina and pedicles align in such a way that the superior articular process approximates with the inferior articular process of the vertebra placed above.

Meninges The three membranes that surround the spinal cord—the dura mater, arachnoid mater and pia mater (Table 5.2). They contain CSF to support the spinal cord.

5.1.2 Spinal Cord

The spinal cord continues from the brain stem at the base of foramen magnum and extends to the conus medullaris which ends between level L1–L2. The cross-section of the spinal cord has a central gray matter while the rest is white matter. The gray

Table 5.2 Meninges

Meninges	Extent	Significance
1. Pia mater	Inferiorly fuses with filum terminale	Innermost meninges
2. Arachnoid mater	Terminates around S2	Distal to conus medullaris, the subarachnoid space expands, forming the lumbar cistern.
3. Dura mater	Foramen magnum to the filum terminale	Allows to pierce nerve roots fuses with the outer connective tissue covering of the nerve, the perineurium

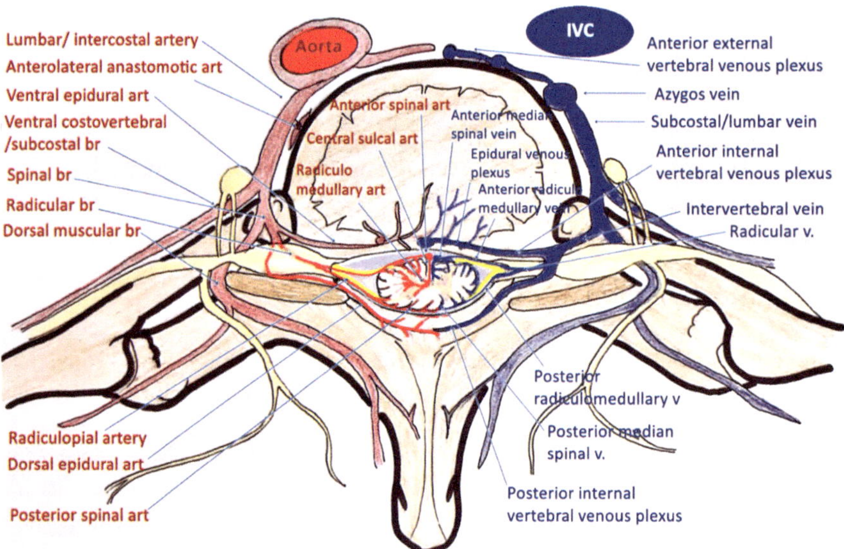

Fig. 5.3 Cross-section of spinal cord with its blood supply

matter is made up of neuroglial cells and neuronal cell bodies while white matter consists of myelinated axons. The dorsal root consists of sensory neurons returning to the spinal cord and also has dorsal root ganglia (DRG). DRG is a collection of cell bodies of the neurons heading back to the cord, while the ventral root consists of motor neurons supplying peripheral organs.

The main blood supply of the spinal cord is from one anterior spinal artery and two posterior spinal arteries (Fig. 5.3). The vertebral arteries pass through the transverse foramen of C1 through C6 and through the foramen magnum to become the basilar artery. The anterior spinal artery from the vertebral artery travels down the spinal cord through anterior sulcus. The ASA provides blood supply to the anterior two-thirds of the spinal cord while the PSA delivers blood to the posterior one-third of the spinal cord.

Both are also supplied with adjuvant arteries, they are segmental arteries to feed both ASA and PSA. Segmental arteries bifurcate to radicular arteries and also give branches such as segmental medullary arteries.

The venous drainage is from anterior and posterior spinal veins. These veins drain to the external venous plexus via the internal venous plexus in epidural space.

The dermatomal supply of the body will help us in deciding the level of neuraxial anaesthesia and whether we can proceed for the desired surgical procedure. The various cutaneous nerves and the dermatomal distribution of the body are illustrated in Fig. 5.4.

There are mainly three types of Neuraxial block which are performed routinely:

1. Subarachnoid Block
2. Epidural
3. Caudal.

The indications and contraindications of the central neuraxial blockade are stated in Table 5.3.

5.2 Physiology of Central Neuraxial Block and Effects on Various System

The central neuraxial blockade affects most of the systems in the body with major effects on the cardiovascular and central nervous systems (Table 5.4). It needs expertise to prevent the complication by anticipating adverse effects and act in a timely manner. Patients may develop symptoms before we can visualise signs on the monitor. The initial period of the block is the time when we need to be extra vigilant and be prepared with optimum preloading/co-loading of fluids and rescue inotropes or vasopressors. The advantage of the epidural blockade is the cardiovascular changes are graded. The subarachnoid blockade has the fastest onset and hence side effects can be seen immediately.

5.2.1 Pharmacology: LA + Adjuvants

The volume required for the subarachnoid block is very less as compared to epidural/caudal anaesthesia. The cerebrospinal fluid (CSF) is in immediate contact with the spinal nerves. It is also observed that CSF may reach up to the level of exit of spinal nerves in the intervertebral foramen. Subarachnoid space is devoid of any barriers such as tough dura mater and hence response of LA is seen within a few minutes compared to epidural/caudal anaesthesia.

LA in SAB comes in direct contact with spinal nerves and sympathetic ganglia.

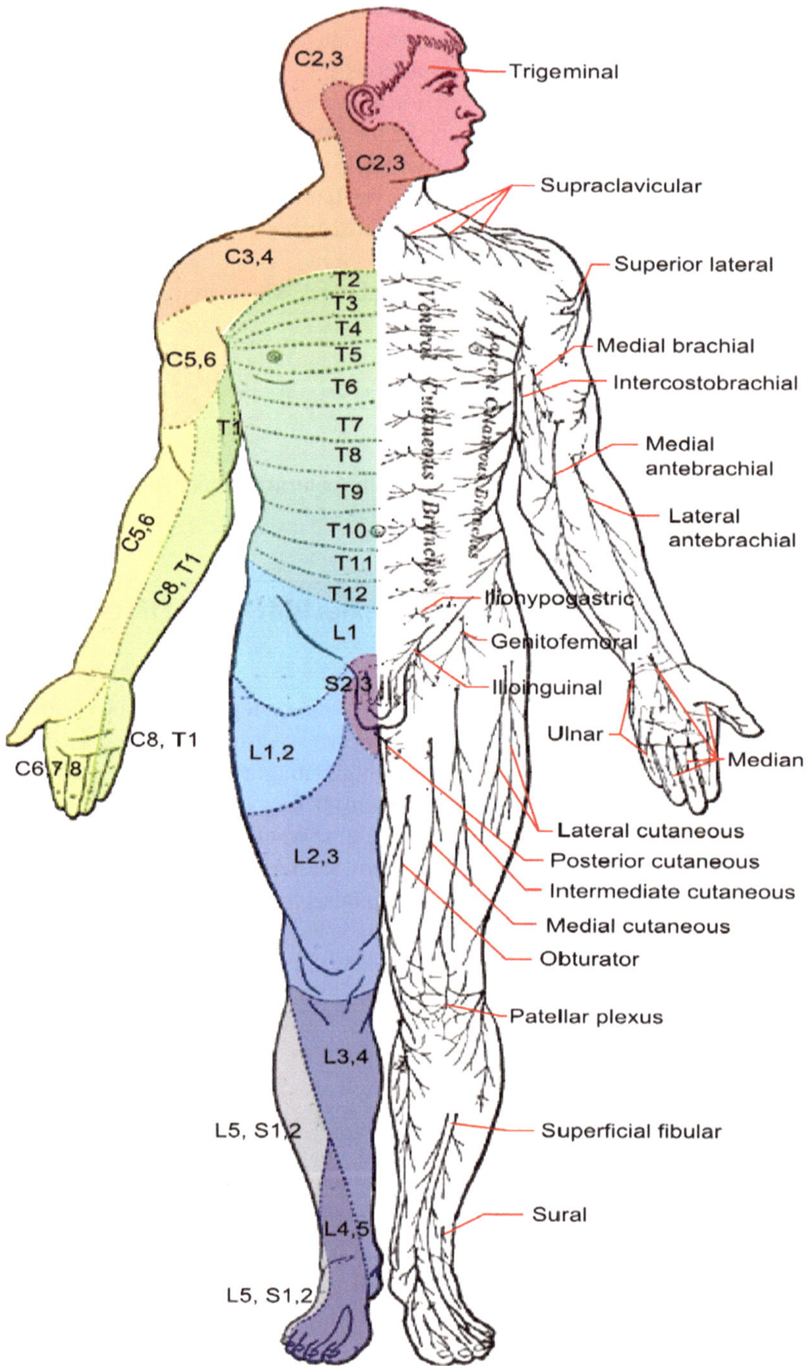

Fig. 5.4 Dermatomes of the body and cutaneous nerves. Resource: *By Mikael Häggström, used with permission.* File:Gray797.png

Table 5.3 Indications and contraindications of CNB

Indications	Contraindications
- Lower limb surgeries - Urological, gynaecological, pelvic surgery. - Obstetric surgeries.	1. ABSOLUTE - Patient refusal - Local infection at the site of intended block. - Raise IOP, Intracranial pathology. - Severe hypotension state. - Allergy to LA.
	2. RELATIVE - Sepsis. - Coagulation disorders - Fixed CO state, e.g. AS - Unable to give consent. - Repair of congenital defect/instrumentation of lower spine.

Table 5.4 Physiological effects of CNB

System	Effects	Clinical implications
1. Cardiovascular	- Severe sympathetic blockade - High spinal also blocks cardioacceleratory fibres - Severe peripheral vasodilatation/ loss of arterial tone	- Hypotension - Bradycardia/tachycardia. - Nausea, vomiting - Shivering
2. Respiratory	- High blockade	Paralysis of respiratory muscles involving cervical nerves. - Dyspnoea
3. GIT	- Sympathetic blockade - Increase in peristalsis. - Intrathecal opioids	- Nausea, vomiting - Ischaemia of the vital abdominal organs.
4. Renal	- Sacral parasympathetic blockade	- Urine retention
5. Central nervous system	- Loss of CSF through dural puncture - Stretching of meninges - Direct needle Trauma to spinal nerves - Lipophilic LA + opoids	- PDPH - Hearing impairment - Permanent neurodeficit of lower limb - Convulsions, respiratory centre depression

5.2.2 Factors Affecting LA Spread

Position of Patient The sitting position of patients tends to provide a higher density of LA to the lower lumbar and sacral segments especially when hyperbaric solutions are used. Whenever patients are allowed to be stabilised in the supine position at the earliest, these effects are minimised. The sitting position seems to be preferred in centers where trained anaesthesia assistants are not available to provide optimal positioning in the lateral approach.

Spinal Level Chosen for the Procedure The apex of the spinal curvature is around the mid lumbar segments (L2–L3) and administration of local anaesthetics in the lower lumbar segments such L4–L5 and below tend to require large volume boluses for epidural anaesthesia to achieve levels above T10. Spinal anaesthetic single shot doses when administered in distal lumbar segments need to be monitored carefully with adjustments in patient positioning such as trendelenburg maneuvers to ensure good sensory levels for cesarean sections.

Choice of LA and Additives The choice of local anaesthetic is chiefly influenced by the presence of glucose to enhance the baricity of the local anaesthetic. This allows for preferential mobility of the local anaesthetics with patient positioning, e.g. Sitting position for saddle block. Hypobaric solutions are largely not in practice and while isobaric solutions are used to minimize shifting of positions and achieve blockade on the side of decubitus position. E.g. Hip fracture with operating side up. Isobaric solutions tend to have longer onset time or perception of the density of blockade in comparison with hyperbaric solutions.

Additives Adjuvant has an important role in enhancing the effect of LA in terms of duration, quality and onset. Opioids are the most frequently used adjuvant. Intrathecal opioid receptors localised in lamina I and II at the spinal dorsal horn reduces nociceptive transmission. The opioids having high lipid solubility and low pKa results in an extremely potent analgesic effect of fast onset but leads to a shorter duration of action. The opioids with low lipid solubility like morphine have slow onset but prolong action and which is also responsible for the cranial spread of the drug [1]. Intrathecal morphine provides 24 h of analgesia. Obstetric patients undergoing cesarean section are more comfortable with 100–200 mcg of intrathecal morphine [2]. Epidural 3 mg of morphine is also sufficient to have the similar effect. Opioids have effects on the central as well as the peripheral nervous system. Other adjuvants studied are buprenorphine, tramadol, dexmedetomidine, clonidine, dexamethasone, ketamine, midazolam, neostigmine. The efficacy and safety are to be considered while selecting any one of them.

Volume of LA Determination of volume of local anaesthetic is dependent on the height of expected sensory blockade to be achieved, the height of the patient. A lower segment caesarian section can be safely performed with local anaesthetic volume ranging from 1.6 ml to 2.5 ml of 0.5% Bupivacaine heavy solution to achieve a level of T6 dermatome.

Spread of LA This denotes the cephalad ascent of the local anaesthesia in spinal anaesthesia as the distal blockade is complete. Epidural anaesthetic is segmental and largely dependent on the volume of injection and the corresponding spread cephalocaudally. The chief determinants seem to be the volume more than the concentration of local anaesthetics. The presence of adiposity in the epidural space from systemic obesity, ossification of lateral spinal foramina results in higher cephalad spread of LA. Lipophilicity of opioids determines the local (fentanyl, lipophilic) versus systemic (morphine, hydrophilic) spread of opioids.

5.2.3 Conduct of Central Neuraxial Blockade: EQUIPMENTS

- Spinal anaesthesia is performed under aseptic precautions. An anaesthesiologist must strictly follow strict asepsis, wear a sterile gown with a sterile pair of gloves. The skin preparation of back can be done either by povidone-iodine or by chlorhexidine. Each of the solutions has its own advantage. Iodine requires 2–3 min of contact time and due to its colour it is easy to identify unprepared areas, while chlorhexidine acts quickly and transparent in colour.
- After sterile preparation of the skin the cleaning solution must be discarded immediately as it may contaminate the spinal needle. There have been incidences of drug errors, where the chlorhexidine was injected intrathecally. Contamination of spinal needles may cause chemical meningitis.
- Operating theatre must be well equipped for general anaesthesia as well. The airway equipments, general anaesthesia and emergency drugs should be made available.
- Intralipid availability and the place where it is usually stored should always be checked along with the expiry. The Local anaesthetic systemic toxicity (LAST) cart should always be checked in the morning while conducting regional anaesthesia.
- Routine monitors as per AAGBI and one large-bore IV cannula is essential before the procedure.
- Depending on the cardiac function, co-loading or preloading of crystalloids should be done as per the department protocol.
- The choice of spinal needle and gauge is individual preference. A small gauge e.g. 27G needle with pencil point causes less chance of PDPH as compared to cutting needles. The pencil point needle requires an introducer before inserting the needle to cut through the ligaments.
- The most commonly preferred needle e.g. in obstetric patients are 27G whitacre needle with introducer.
- The epidural needle commonly used are 16/18G Tuohy needle with marking upto 9 cm on needle shaft (Table 5.5).

Table 5.5 Spinal needles

Needle	Description
1. Pencil point - Whitacre - Sprotte	- Non cutting, round tip. - Opening is 3–4 mm proximal to the tip of needle
2. Cutting needle - Quincke's	- Sharp tip, short bevel
3. Combined spinal epidural	- Usually fine gauge pencil point needle through tuohy epidural needles

5.2.4 Position and Approach

- The position of the patient during the spinal anaesthesia depends on the anaesthesiologist's preference and patient comfort.
- The sitting position is better while palpating landmarks of the spine. The lumbar curvature minimises sudden cephalad spread of the drug when the patient is asked to lie supine. The lumbar dural sac is known to be distended maximally in the sitting position
- The lateral position is comfortable for the patient but may need assistance to stabilise the shoulder and pelvis, preventing rotation of the spine. This curling back or 'universal flexion' or 'fetal position' may open up intervertebral spaces.
- The lumbar spine gets straightened in the lateral position, more chances of the cephalad spread of drugs are seen.

5.2.5 Complications of CNB

1. Hemodynamics changes
   (a) Hypotension
   (b) Bradycardia
   (c) Cardiac arrest
   (d) Supine hypotension in gravid patients
2. Respiration and apnea and complications in respiratory disease
   (a) Increased secretions
   (b) Brocho spasm—sympathetic blockade and unapposed parasympathetic actions
   (c) No support from accessory muscle—altered mechanics of breathing
   (d) Inability to generate good cough
3. Nerve injury
   (a) Neuropraxia
   (b) Neurotmesis
   (c) Axonotmesis
4. Spinal and epidural haematoma
5. Residual neuropraxia
6. Cauda equina

5.2.6 Advantages of Central Neuraxial Nerve Blockade

1. Good quality of pain relief in intraoperative and postoperative phase
2. Reduced systemic stress response: humoral and autonomic effects
3. Reduced risk of deep vein thrombosis and subsequent pulmonary embolism

4. Enhanced surgical operating conditions: improved microvasculature and anastomosis improved bowel mesenteric blood flow and immobility
5. Reduced postoperative nausea and vomiting (PONV): reduced opioid consumption, improved bowel motility, reduced bowel distention
6. Enhanced postoperative respiratory function: early ambulation, better participation in chest physiotherapy and ability to cough, minimal restriction of diaphragmatic excursions and hence reduced chance of basal atelectasis

5.2.7 Sonoanatomical Guidance

- Ultrasonography is widely applied in identifying the neuraxial space. It has become routine in many institutions to have a scout scan of the lower back pre-procedure or atleast have an ultrasonography machine standby before attempting a block. Real-time needle manipulation while performing neuraxial block can be done, however it is a bit inconvenient and time-consuming [3].
- Some anaesthesiologists prefer to mark the spaces and identify the epidural depth with USG before attempting a difficult neuraxial block e.g. in obese patients/obstetric cases/scoliosis/osteophytic spine patients where landmarks are difficult to palpate [4].
- Ultrasonography along with fluoroscopy has been routinely used for chronic pain procedures and definitely decreases the chances of radiation exposure [5].
- Recently many authors have published the usefulness of USG in obstetric anaesthesia as the obesity obscures marking and also helps in decreasing the attempts and improves analgesia.
- Routine scanning before the procedure also establishes a quick learning curve for residents and allows the anaesthesiologist to apply sound knowledge of USG in difficult cases.
- The ergonomics also plays an important role as it reduces operators' fatigue and improves comfort while performing the block.

5.3 Ultrasonography of Central Neuraxial Space

Preparation A curvilinear probe of frequency 2–5 MHz is preferred to cover a wider area over back. The probe should be covered with sterile sheets under aseptic technique depending on the instituition protocol. USG probe can be covered by two large transparent films (perpendicular to each other) and hub along with the cord should be draped with the sterile sheets. Camera cover used in laparoscopy is also being widely used.

Position Patient can be positioned in sitting, lateral or prone depending on the procedure and patient comfort.

Orientation The idea of checking the orientation marker is to know the point of needle entry. The probe should be placed craniocaudal and marker facing the cranial side. This should be routinely done when you first hold the probe for any of the regional block i.e. to orient yourself with the orientation marker. It should be fixed in your head before performing any block so that you do not struggle halfway in search of anatomical structure while doing the procedure.

Ultrasonography Window The ultrasound waves cannot penetrate bones and produces what is known as black acoustic window. So there are two places which act as a window for us to visualise the neuraxial structure. First is *interspinous space* while doing the transverse scan with USG. Second is the *interlaminar space* on the paramedian sagittal scan.

5.3.1 USG Probe Placement

The above-mentioned planes (Fig. 5.5) are used commonly to find the acoustic window of the spinal cord. The basic definitions of the planes will help in describing them better.

1. Transverse plane: A horizontal plane that is parallel to the ground and perpendicular to the coronal plane. It divides the body into upper and lower parts.
2. Coronal plane: A vertical lane perpendicular to the ground and at right angles to the sagittal plane dividing the body into anterior and posterior parts.
3. Median plane: A longitudinal plane that passes through the midline of the body dividing the body into right and left half.
4. Saggital plane: A longitudinal plane that is parallel to the median plane.

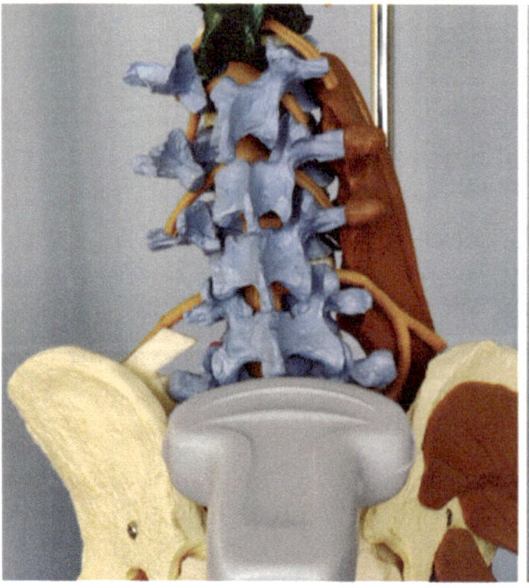
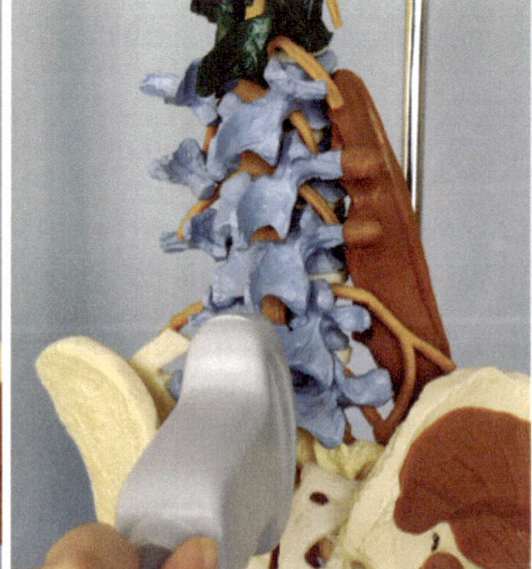

Fig. 5.5 Scanning technique of the ultrasound image of the spine: Left: transverse scan, Right: Sagittal scan

Start with scanning the sacral area identify the lumbosacral region and then count and advance the usg probe cranially. The first gap after sacrum is L5–S1 space. Other spaces can be counted from this (Fig. 5.6).

1. *Transverse Scan*

The transverse plane is horizontal plane parallel to the ground. The USG probe is placed over the spinous process (Fig. 5.7). The probe is then gradually slid over to the interspinous space to get the clear view of dura. When the probe is placed over the spinous process, the hyperechoic structure of the spinous process obscures the neuraxial space. This may not be helpful to see neuraxial structures but its definitive guide that the probe is centrally placed over the midline. The transverse scan visualises the spinous process and its acoustic shadow.

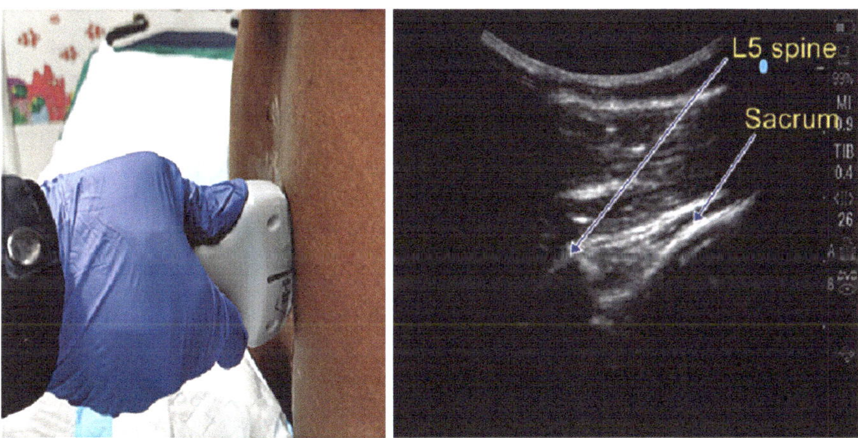

Fig. 5.6 Identification of the lumbar space with the help of L5–S1 interspace

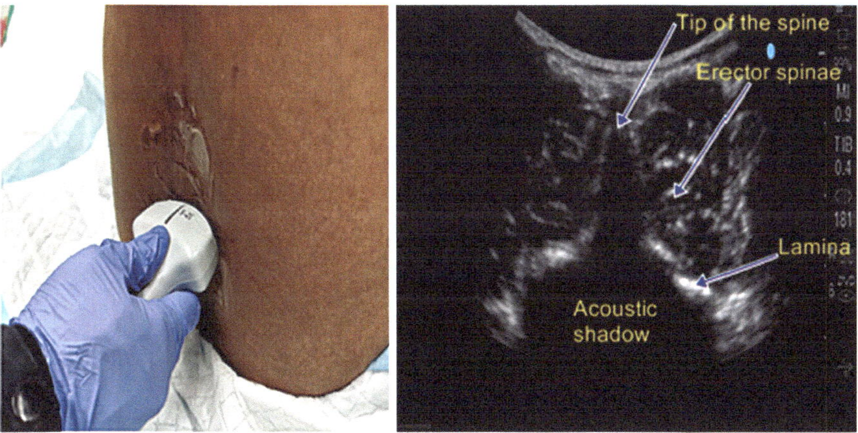

Fig. 5.7 Transverse scan at the level of the spinous process

The transverse interspinous view needs s alignment of USG waves which is achieved with the tilt of the probe either upwards or downwards (Fig. 5.8). The structures visualised are posterior dura with epidural space. A black window filled with fluid/CSF is intrathecal space. It is also possible to visualise anterior dura which is hyperechoic structure. The acoustic shadow of the articular process (AP) is seen bilaterally which gives the appearance of *'cat's head sign' or bat's wing sign.*

2. *Sagittal Scan*

The sagittal plane is the longitudinal plane in the midline (Fig. 5.9). The probe is placed on a sagittal plane. This is done to mark the point of entry. The skin marking is also done from transverse scan.

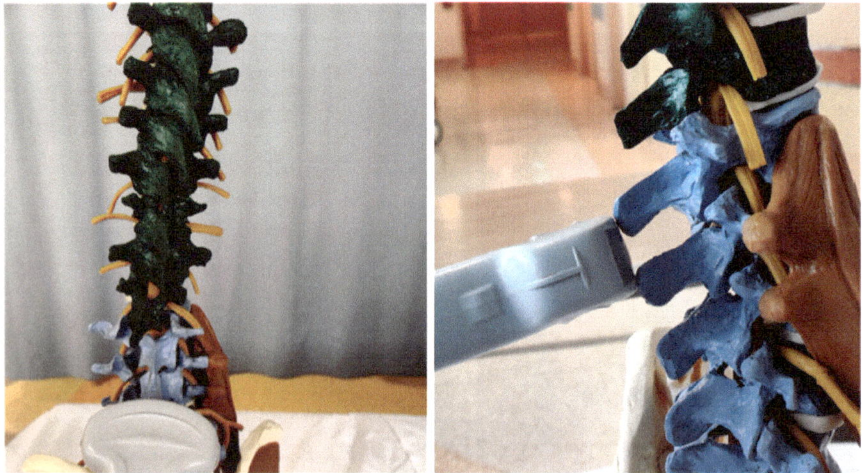

Fig. 5.8 Transverse scan at the interspinous process level

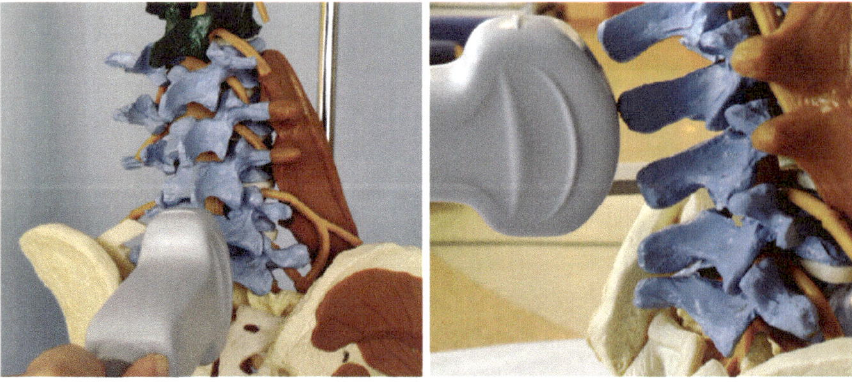

Fig. 5.9 Sagittal plane of obtaining the longitudinal view of the spine

In this way, a midpoint is chosen by drawing the lines in both the planes. For real-time needle placement, the paramedian sagittal oblique (PMSO) view is preferred where the probe is tilted medially while on sagittal plane.

The technique of moving the probe from sagittal plane to parasagittal plane is shown in Fig. 5.10. The usg probe placed in craniocaudal orientation on the lamina, articular process and then on transverse process.

At this level, it is possible to see neuraxial structures. In the interlaminar gap, can see the ligamentum flavum, dura as a hyperechoic structure. Anterior to dura is subarachnoid space filled with CSF, appears hypoechoic. Sometimes hyperechoic anterior dura may be visualised.

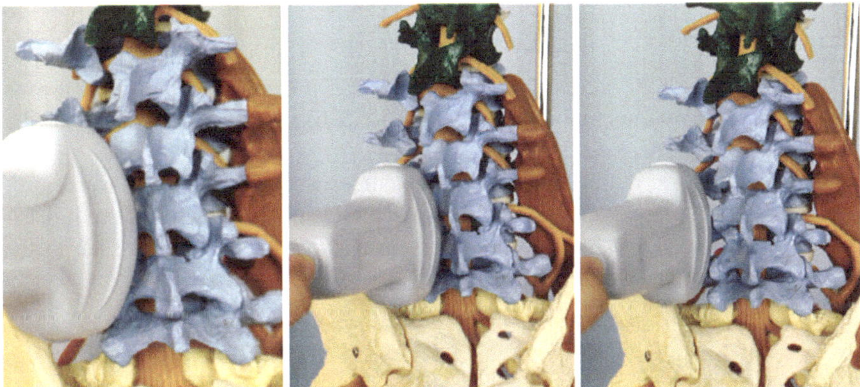

Fig. 5.10 Scanning technique for moving the probe from sagittal to parasagittal area. We can see the lamina, appears hyperechoic and looks like the head and neck of horse, called as *'horse head sign'* (Fig. 5.11)

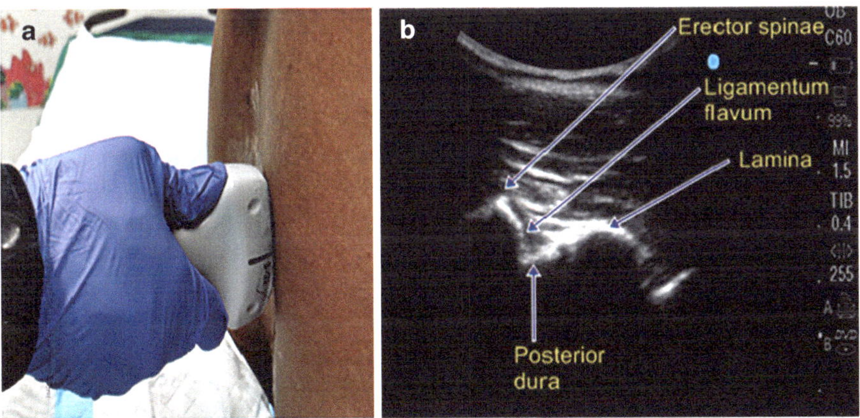

Fig. 5.11 (**a** and **b**) Saggital scan at the lamina

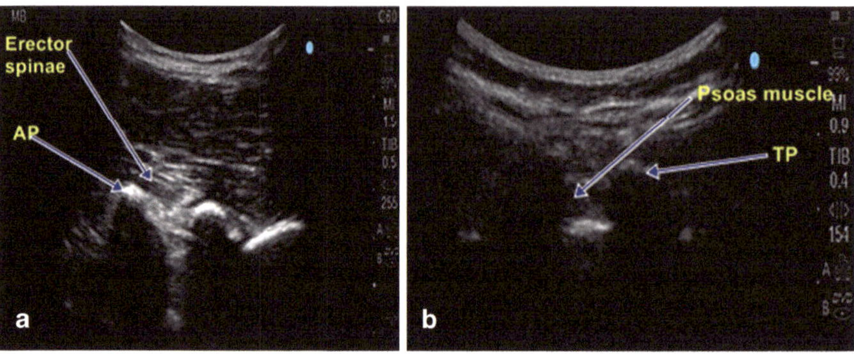

Fig. 5.12 Paramedian saggital scan—(**a**) at the level of the articular process (AP) and (**b**) transverse process (TP)

As we move probe laterally over the articular processes, hyperechoic waves appear without any intervening gaps, described as like a camel hump and called a *'camel hump sign'* (Fig. 5.12a).

Further lateral to the articular processes comes in view of the transverse processes (TP). They appear small round hyperechoic structures also referred as trident. Since these finger-like projections appear as a trident which is seen in the hands of Lord Shiva (Fig. 5.12b).

5.4 Blockmate Pearls

1. *Incomplete or Inadequate Spinal Anaesthesia*

   This is common when adequate level of spinal anaesthesia is not obtained to the desired heights (eg T4 for cesarean sections surgeries) and it is not dense enough to achieve all components of central neuraxial blockade.

   - In spite of the best efforts, it is difficult to get the desired response in many cases.
   - Ideal is to explain the patient all the above possible outcome{it is not uncommon to have failed spinal} beforehand and then proceed with the block. Theatre should be adequately prepared for general anaesthesia.
   - It is in spite of the desired action, the patient is not satisfied due to intact sensation from unaffected part of the abdomen. This may cause excessive anxiety. The decision to administer sedation to allay anxiety after confirming the level of anaesthesia must be individualised.
   - A structured systematic approach for the management of a spinal anaesthetic is shown in Fig. 5.13.

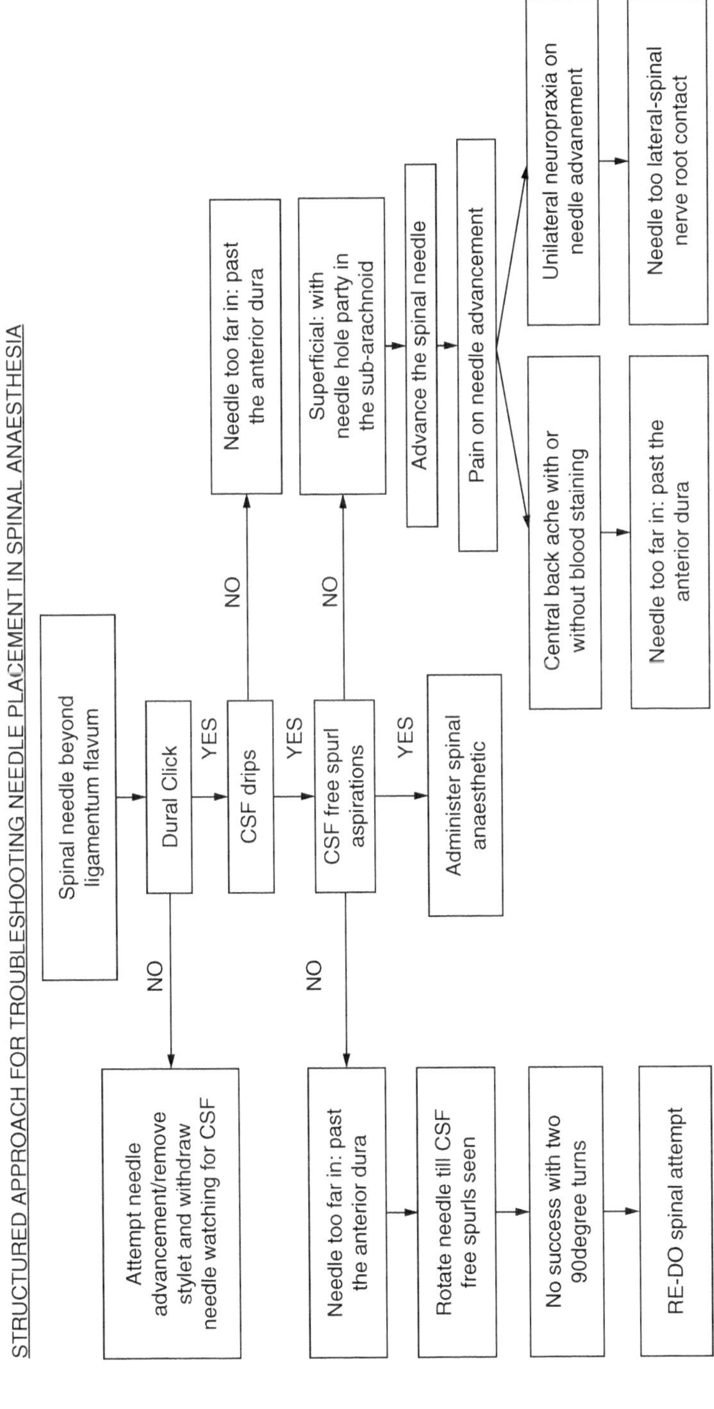

Fig. 5.13 Flow chart for systematic approach in troubleshooting spinal anaesthesia

Structured Approach for Troubleshooting Needle Placement in Spinal Anaesthesia

2. *Difficult Spinal Techniques*

   Procedural difficulty with spinal anaesthesia is related to modifiable factors such as patient anxiety (consider sedation), suboptimal patient positioning (qualified support staff, shifting from sitting to lateral or vice versa) and from innate anatomical difficulties. These include excessive lumbar lordosis, kyphoscoliosis, ossified interspinous ligaments and reactive arthritis of the back (ankylosing spondylosis) with limitations. Most of these conditions can be effectively managed by adequate preoperative mapping of the spinal column with surface and ultrasound-guided mapping of the anatomic landmarks. Scoliosis is best approached from the convex side of the curve as the spaces are wider in that angle. Rest of conditions of the spine are chiefly managed with proficiency in the paramedian approach to needle advancements with access to the midline beyond the ligaments that are potentially ossified.

   Lower lumbar disc-related neuropraxias need to be examined preoperatively and pre-existing deficits should be meticulously documented before central neuraxial blockade is to be attempted. While most of the lumbar or lower back ache seem to be in the L4–S1 segments, the central neuraxial blockade in the L2–L3 and L3–L4 spaces can be feasible.

   Patients with spinal instrumentations need to be evaluated with radiological images for the extent of placement of implants and rods. Instrumentation above L2 is generally safer and while there are reports to suggest safety of performing epidural anaesthesia in patients with lower lumbar instrumentations with ultrasound guidance. The potential concerns are accidental tethering or adhesions resulting in high risk of dural puncture and risk of contamination of the infected spinal prosthesis from the infusions through the catheters.

3. *Intra procedural management of accidental large-bore needle dural puncture (LDP) and Intrathecal catheter:*

   Fig. 5.14. The administration of lumbar epidural analgesia can be challenging especially when it is done with the pressure of time in a pregnant patient having active labour. The frequent sustained contractions of the uterus can result in engorgement of the epidural vessels and results in dynamic changes in pressure and volume of the dural sac. The inability to stay still during contractions and sudden movements after the contraction wane off results in higher chances for an accidental lumbar dural puncture (LDP) with large-bore tuohy needles.

   The flow diagram describes an intraprocedural decision-making process when there is an active 'gush' of CSF with the epidural needle in place or when epidural technique is largely uneventful and yet there is an inadvertent intrathecal catheter placement. When there is a large volume CSF leak as in the first case, it requires a quick decision-making process to avoid further fluid loss. Whether the plan is to abandon the procedure or to re-site the epidural catheter in another

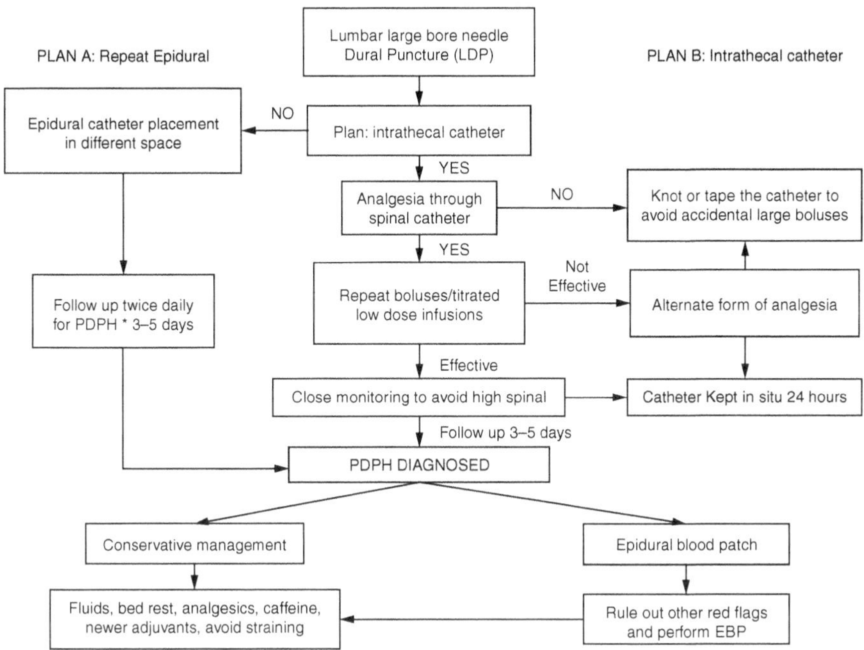

Fig. 5.14 Flow chart for Large dural needle puncture. *PDPH* post-dural puncture headache, *EBP* epidural blood patch

space, the tuohy needle removal needs to be achieved only after placing the stylette back into the needle. This is performed to push the dura back to avoid an encored dural sleeve. This happens because of the drag of the dura towards the epidural space theoretically making the orifice larger resulting in higher chances for leak.

Where the practice is to achieve partial 'seal' of the large hole, threading of the epidural catheter is achieved into the intrathecal space and keeping it in situ for 24 h for the formation of fine fibrin mesh. A recent review showed that there is no consensus on what is the best course of action (whether to place an intrathecal catheter) for reducing the incidence of post-dural puncture headache (PDPH) or achieve positive epidural pressure through continuous epidural infusion that can potentially minimise CSF leaks through purges during strong uterine contraction.

The PDPH is a result of low intracranial pressure. The frontotemporal pain is because of dural traction. The management is chiefly conservative with bed rest, avoidance of anti-gravity posturing, fluid hydrations, oral analgesics and caffeine to modify the vascular tone. If conservative measures are not effective and activities of daily life are compromised, an epidural blood patch (EBP) with 15–40 ml of patient's own blood is recommended with a success rate of >90%.

Placing an intrathecal catheter is an individual anaesthetist's preference. The ideal is to place an intrathecal catheter for inadvertent large needle dural puncture and keep for atleast 24 h to decrease the incidence of headache. An institute should make a guideline to avoid possible miscommunication between the staff and anaesthesiologist. Steps to follow when managing an unplanned intrathecal catheter are illustrated in Fig. 5.15 [6]

(a) *Thread Catheter:* The moment you see gush of CSF coming through the tuohy needle , the epidural catheter is threaded to the intrathecal space.
(b) *Confirm:* There are ways to confirm that fluid aspirated is CSF. A simple test of raising the height of the catheter, will not show a meniscus sign. Testing the fluid for glucose, protein with the rapid sticks.
(c) *Label:* Appropriate labelling of 'Intrathecal catheter' at multiple sites. Filter, Infusion system, LA fluid bag all need to label appropriately as 'Intrathecal catheter' with unique colour.
(d) *Communicate:* Patient and relatives should be informed about it immediately and known complications should be discussed with them. It is recommended to keep the catheter for 24 h. Communicate with the fellow anaesthesiologist who will be attending the patient. Ward staff should be communicated regarding the catheter. An anaesthesiologist will follow-up 24 h later to remove the catheter should be mentioned in bold letters in files. Meanwhile staff and patient should inform anaesthesiologist immediately if the patient develops neurodeficit, headache, backache.
(e) *Follow-up:* PDPH usually develops 24–48 h post-procedure. It is manageable by oral analgesics. Frequent follow-up might be needed.

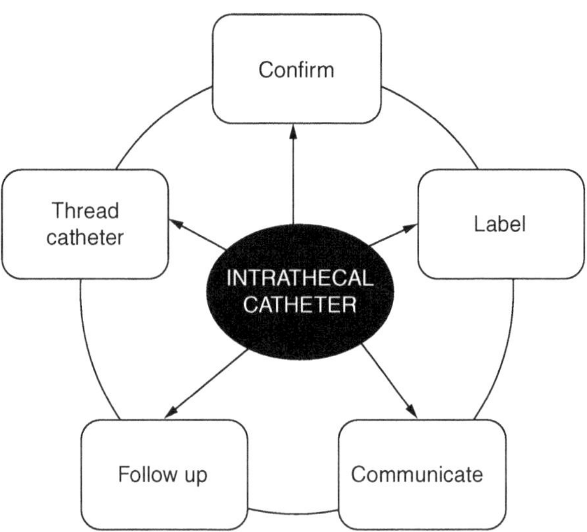

Fig. 5.15 Intrathecal catheter management

4. *Anterior Spinal Artery Syndrome:*
   The acute ASA syndrome is characterized by bilateral flaccid paresis or plegia below the lesion level, loss of motor reflexes, and dissociated sensory loss. Most common causes are persistent intraoperative hypotension, vascular disease causing obstruction to the blood flow.
5. *Cauda Equina Syndrome(CES):*
   It is a neurological complication following a central neuraxial block, complicated by neurodeficit of lower limb, bladder and bowel involvement. Trauma, infection, hematoma, intrathecal catheter with LA infusion are few of the direct causes of the syndrome. The nerves are usually unmyelinated resembles horse's tail, which has more risk of developing nerve damage. Treating the patient as early as within 48 h after the onset of the syndrome provides a significant advantage
6. *Backache:*
   Chronic backache history will suggest some stretching of muscle, joints or ligaments of the lower back. Severe pain may arise from impinged nerves from a slipped disc. Discs acts as a cushion for the vertebra. Any annulus tear may lead to herniation of the discs. The neurological deficit may occur due to this. Anaesthesiologist must do a detailed neurological examination and document it before giving any kind of central neuraxial block.
7. *Multiple Sclerosis:*
   Multiple sclerosis is an automimmune disorder affecting the nervous system. It adds inflammation and destruction of the neuronal myelin sheath. The incidences are more seen in young women. An anasthesiologist may come across obstetric women affected by MS during cesarean delivery or labour analgesia. The risk of neuropathy in already damaged nerves is 0.4% [7] due to the phenomenon called as 'double crush sydrome'. Also demyelinated neurons delay the conduction. Since obstetric patients having difficult airway and fear of losing airway is more catastrophic than transient neurological symptoms in the lower limb, regional remains the first choice for many parturients. General anaesthesia leads to foetal exposure of opioids and other IV induction agents. The decision to place a central neuraxial block should be made by involving patient, obstetrician, paediatrician and neurologist where the patient is following-up.
8. *Tattoo:*
   During the tattooing process, the needles penetrate the epidermis, and the pigment is deposited along the entire needle tract. After healing the pigment is engulfed by marcophages and excreted in lymphatics. Th pigment left in loose fibrous tissues gives the colour. Anaesthesiologist are concerned over lower back tattoos as while giving a central neuraxial block the pigment may get transferred to the CSF and may cause infection,inflammation, neuropathy and meningitis. There has been suggestion to give a nick on the skin before inserting any needle to the neuraxial space [8].

   A structured approach for troubleshooting a epidural central neruaxial blockade is shown in Fig. 5.16.

Structured Approach for Troubleshooting Needle Placement in Epidural Anaesthesia

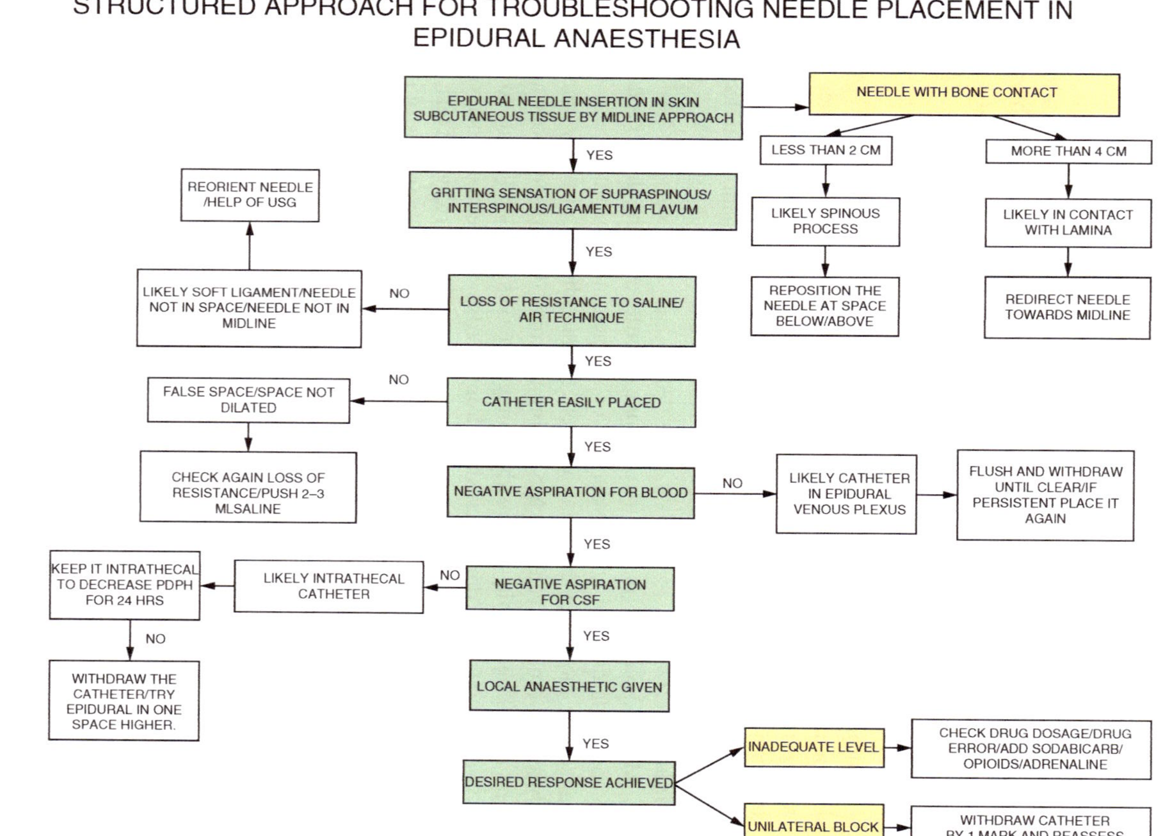

Fig. 5.16 Structured approach for troubleshooting epidural anaesthesia

5.4.1 Caudal Anaesthesia

5.4.1.1 Applied Anatomy

- Caudal anaesthesia is being used widely in the paediatric population due to the easy accessibility of caudal space. Anesthesiologist not well versed with this technique also prefers other superficial blocks like ilioinguinal, penile, etc.
- Recently due to advancements in the pain speciality, the caudal block has gained its popularity in treating backache, chronic pain by using fluoroscopy and ultrasonography.
- Anatomy of caudal space is all about understanding Sacrum.
- Superior surface: Wide and articulates with L5 vertebra forms lumbosacral joint. Sometimes we may come across sacralization of the lumbar vertebra as well as lumbarization of sacrum.
- Anterior surface: Concave in shape.
- Posterior surface: Convex with fused spinous processes defined as median crest. Spinal nerves exit through the intervertebral foramina.
- *Sacral Hiatus*: Sacrum is simply fused five sacral vertebra. When the S5 lamina and spinous process fails to fuse in the midline exposing the sacral canal marks the opening of caudal space. This opening is also called as sacral hiatus.
- *Sacral Cornua*: The remnant of the inferior articular surface of S5 marks the cornua, bony landmark of the space.
- *Caudal space* can be imagined as an equilateral triangle. The base is made up of bilateral posterior superior iliac crest and the apex denotes the cornua (Fig. 5.17).
- Ligamentum flavum continues as sacrococcygeal ligament which covers the space. The give way of this ligament is essential for the block. The give way of sacrococcygeal ligament is similar to give way of ligamentum flavum in lumbar epidural.

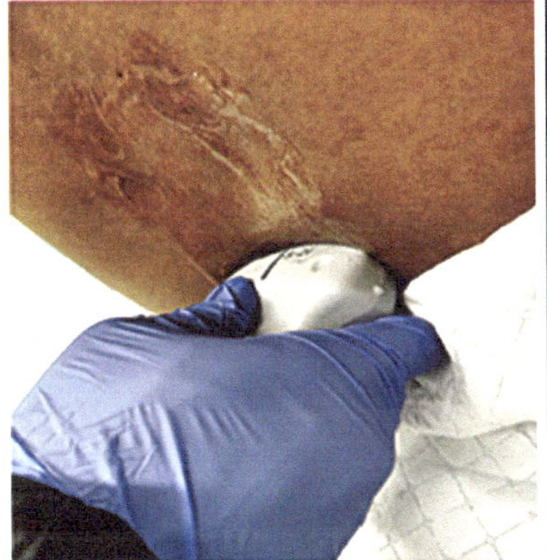

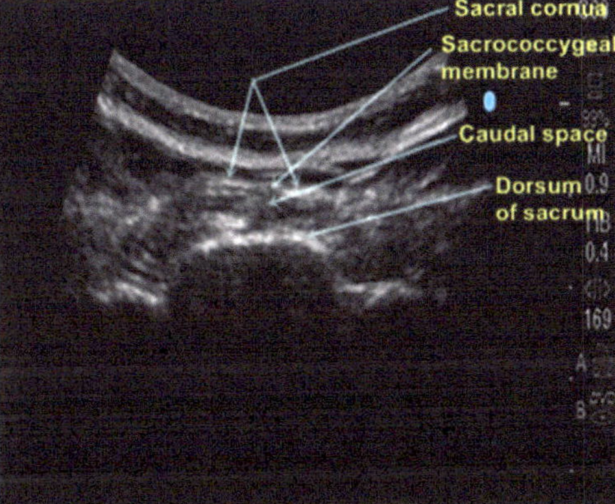

Fig. 5.17 USG for caudal space: Left: probe holding in the transverse plane, Right: Transverse scan of the caudal space showing the sonoanatomy landmarks

5.4.2 Needling Technique

- Caudal block is performed after turning the child in a decubitus position with the knee drawn to the chest, safeguarding the airway either by holding the mask or by inserting a definitive airway and allowing for spontaneous or assisted ventilation.
- Adults can remain awake and a prone position is preferred.Pillow is placed at the lower abdomen to flex the lower lumbar vertebra.
- Clean the skin with antiseptic solution and drape the desired area. The solution must not touch the anal mucosa, may have irritant effects.
- The most palpable landmark is sacral cornua often described as dimple, midpoint can be in line with the natal cleft.
- The needle choice of gauge is as per the age, height and pad of fat.
- The most common needle gauge is 21G, 25G varying in length. 22G hypodermic needle is commonly used with a short bevel to get the best feel of tissue. Adult caudal block is performed with a spinal needle ranging from 22G to 25G. Very fine needles may bend during the placement of caudal injection hence to be avoided.

5.5 Blockmate Pearls

- Failure to identify caudal space due to impalpable sacral cornua may lead to block failure. We will suggest to use ultrasonography as it is easily available in the operating area, to be used while performing the procedure. This also gives a real-time image of local anaesthetic during injection.
- Accidental dural puncture is a potential complication of the caudal block. Dura usually ends at S3 level. Anatomical variants where sacrum is not fused at higher level may raise the sacral hiatus which brings the point of needle insertion close to the dura. Caudal injection should be avoided in this case, otherwise may lead to inadvertent spinal anaesthesia.
- Adjuvants like opioids should be used with caution as paediatric patients are more prone to respiratory depression.
- Adequate dose of LA is important to achieve the desired level during surgery.

5.5.1 What Will You Do? (Table 5.6) [9]

Table 5.6 Troubleshooting for caudal anaesthesia

1. Give way/first pop	Needle to be directed 30 degrees to the skin and advance a few mm into sacral canal.
2. Encounter bone immediately	Usually anterior wall of sacrum, withdraw slightly and decrease the angle.
3. Subcutaneous bulging	Needle needs to be advanced further as it still has not pierced sacrococcygeal ligament.
4. CSF on aspiration	After confirming clear continuous free flow of fluid, the procedure should be abandoned.
5. Blood on aspiration.	Withdraw needle completely and begin the procedure from the start.
6. Bradycardia/tachycardia	Caudal needs to be done in controlled environment with available resuscitation equipment. Bradycardia: Stop injecting. Consider accidental dural puncture and high spinal anaesthesia from large volume injection. Apnea, pupillary dilatations and bradycardia are common. Tachycardia: Possible intravascular placement. Tachycardia can happen when giving test dose of Lignocaine + Adrenaline. As aspiration tests are not foolproof.
7. Encounter wide bony surface after advancing the needle more than 15 mm.	Needle may not be in the midline and might be hitting sacral lamina. Need to withdraw needle completely and find the midline spot of insertion
8. No Pop inspite of being in midline and using adequate length of needle.	Entry point could have been far from SCL in coccyx region.
9. Unilateral block	Post operatively may be assessed as weakness over one leg as compared to other. LA is deposited unilaterally. Needle might have been directed on one side after piercing SCL or falsely depositing LA directly over sacral foramina.

References

1. Hindle A. Intrathecal opioids in the management of acute postoperative pain. Contin Educ Anaesth Crit Care Pain. 2008;8:81–5.
2. Girgin NK, Gurbet A, Turker G, Aksu H, Gulhan N. Intrathecal morphine in anaesthesia for cesarean delivery: dose–response relationship for combinations of low dose intrathecal morphine and spinal bupivacaine. J Clin Anaesth. 2008;20:180–5.
3. Chin KJ, Karmakar MK, Peng P. Ultrasonography of the adult thoracic and lumbar spine for central neuraxial blockade. Anaesthesiology. 2011;114:1459–85. https://doi.org/10.1097/ALN.0b013e318210f9f8.
4. Jain K, Puri A, Taneja R, Jaiswal A, Jain A. Preprocedural ultrasound as an adjunct to blind conventional technique for epidural neuraxial blockade in patients undergoing hip or knee joint replacement surgery: a randomised controlled trial. Indian J Anaesth. 2019;63(11):924–31. https://doi.org/10.4103/ija.IJA_327_19.
5. Wu T, Zhao WH, Dong Y, Song HX, Li JH. Effectiveness of ultrasound guided versus fluoroscopy or computed tomography scanning guidance in lumbar facet joint injections in adults with facet joint syndrome: a meta-analysis of controlled trials. Arch Phys Med Rehabil. 2016;97(9):1558–63. https://doi.org/10.1016/j.apmr.2015.11.013.
6. Rupasinghe M. Guidelines for insertion of intrathecal/spinal catheter following unintended dural puncture. APSF Newsletter Winter. 2013–2014;28(3):73.
7. O'Neal MA, Chang L. Postpartum spinal cord, roots, plexus and peripheral nerve injuries involving the lower extremities: a practical approach. Anaesth Analg. 2015;120(1):141–8.
8. Douglas MJ, Swenerton JE. Epidural anaesthesia in three parturients with lumbar tattoos: a review of possible implications. Can J Anaesth. 2003;49(10):1057–60. https://doi.org/10.1007/BF03017902.
9. Raux O, Dadure C, Carr J, Rochette A, capdevila X. Pediatric caudal anaesthesia. Anaesthesia. 2010;26:32–6.

6 Paediatric Regional Anaesthesia

S. Sanjay Prabhu and Arunangshu Chakraborty

6.1 Introduction

Regional anaesthesia has become an integral part of paediatric anaesthesia. The benefits on regional anaesthesia in paediatrics include:

1. To achieve an opioid-free anaesthetic technique, as opioid usage leads to more troublesome side effects [e.g. Nausea and Vomiting].
2. Potential reduction in the incidence of persistent post-surgical pain [PPSP].
3. Decrease requirement for anaesthetic agents leads to lower incidence and severity of emergence delirium.
4. Though the concept of anaesthesia related neurotoxicity has been challenged recently, it might still be useful to minimise exposure to general anaesthetic agents during longer procedures.
5. Physiological reasons suggest that children do have a lower pain threshold, particularly younger children [up to the age of 1 year]. Poorly developed descending inhibitory pathways leads to abnormal spinal modulation of pain. This results in increased pain perception and allodynia [non-noxious stimuli perceived as painful]. So effective regional analgesia can significantly reduce the consequences of pain.

Large surveys also suggest that the complication rate is low [1]. Ultrasound guidance (USG) is increasingly being recommended and used in children, though a recent large multicentre observational study reports that USG is used only in 23% of all regional techniques [2].

S. S. Prabhu (✉)
Apollo Children's Hospital, Chennai, India

A. Chakraborty
Department of Anaesthesia, CC and Pain, Tata Medical Center, Kolkata, India

A. Chakraborty (ed.), *Blockmate*, https://doi.org/10.1007/978-981-15-9202-7_6

6.1.1 How Is USGRA Different in Children and What Are Its Benefits?

1. USG has made new peripheral nerve blocks possible (favoured over central neuraxial blocks) and made older blocks safer.
2. Most regional techniques in children are done under general anaesthesia. Symptoms of Local anaesthetic systemic toxicity (LAST) and symptoms related to needle-related nerve injury are masked. These are minimised by USG guided techniques.
3. USG enables real-time imaging of structures, needle movement, needle trajectory and spread of injectate. This increases the success rate, minimises complications, decreases the dosage of LA and accelerates the onset of the block.
4. Neuraxial structures are better visualised in children compared to adults due to incomplete ossification.
5. Due to smaller and superficial structures—Linear probe will suffice for most blocks.
6. Requires more precision and dexterity due to the smaller size of children, particularly children less than 2 years.
7. Smaller footprint probes will be required for children <10 kg.

6.1.2 Ultrasound Probe Characteristics and Imaging

Most blocks in children can be done with the linear probe. Due to the relatively superficial depth at which structures are present.

A useful first approximation for estimating a depth of penetration (dp) for a given frequency is dp = 60/f cm-MHz, where f is given in megahertz.

1. Linear probe (6–13 MHz), Depth up to 6 cm.
2. Hockey stick probe (6–13 MHz) has a smaller footprint and is used for very small children or in places where the linear probe is too big to achieve complete contact with the skin.
3. Curvilinear probe (3–8 MHz) is advisable for deeper blocks in older children [Sciatic nerve, Lumbar plexus].
4. Imaging technique—Children require a shorter depth setting and smaller needles.

6.1.3 Clinical Pearls While Doing a USGRA

1. Short bevel needle is useful for two reasons:
   a. To appreciate the loss of resistance through fascial planes.
   b. Less risk of nerve impalement.
2. When using small diameter needles, it is useful to nick the skin with a sharper needle before inserting the actual block needle to prevent the encoring of skin.
3. In small children use an extension tubing between the needle and syringe. This will minimise movement of needle during the injection.

4. Prime the needle with saline— this serves three purposes.
   a. To avoid air affecting the USG images.
   b. For hydro localisation.
   c. To minimise wastage of LA till the actual target is reached.
5. If possible, keep the patient breathing spontaneously to alert for intravascular or subarachnoid injections.
6. Monitor ECG to detect any T wave or ST segment changes that will alert towards intravascular injection.

6.1.4 Prerequisites for Practicing USGRA

1. Learn the basics of USG machine and the probes specific for each block and age of the child.
2. A good knowledge of anatomy is essential and be aware of anatomical variations and physiological differences in children compared to adults (Table 6.1).
3. Know your dosages and select equipment [needles, extension tubing tailored to the age and weight of the child. (Table 6.1).

Table 6.1 Clinical pearls: physiology/pharmacology of LA

Anatomy/physiology	Pharmacological implication
Incomplete myelination	Lesser concentration of LA required
Nerves have a smaller diameter, closer nodes of Ranvier	Lesser concentration of LA required, rapid onset of block
Low protein binding [Alpha 1 acid glycoprotein and albumin] and decreased intrinsic clearance	Increased risk of LAST
Increased volume of distribution in neonates and small infants	Bolus doses cause a lower plasma concentration, but continuous infusions have a potential for toxicity due to slower metabolism and clearance
Immature liver metabolism—cytochrome systems maturing at varying rates: the CYP3A4 within the first 9 months of life compared to the CYP1A2, which can take until 8 years of age to mature	Slower metabolism and longer time for clearance→Increased risk of LAST
Relatively high cardiac output	Accelerates absorption from tissues leading to shorter duration of action, higher initial plasma concentration and hence increased risk of LAST
Higher heart rate in younger children	Increased susceptibility of cardiac toxicity [3]
The clearance of drugs is decreased in those less than 3 months of age, gradually reaching adult levels by 8 months of age	Elimination half-lives of LA are longer in neonates and infants compared to adults
Immature BBB	Higher risk of Neurotoxicity
Loose epidural fat	Higher spread of LA when injected in the caudal space. Epidural catheter can be easily threaded to a higher level [from the caudal route]

6.1.5 Principles of Dosing

- Use a lower concentration of LA.
- Draw up only the pre-calculated dose based on age, weight and comorbidities (Table 6.2).
- Levobupivacaine or Ropivacaine are preferred over other LA [better cardiovascular safety profile and less motor blockade].
- In blocks where a higher volume is required [fascial plane blocks, bilateral blocks and when a higher level needs to be achieved as in trying to get a dermatomal block to the upper abdomen with a caudal block] it is pertinent that a dilute concentration of LA is used. A volume of 0.5 ml/kg will generally cover most interfacial plane blocks.
- In USG guided nerve blocks where nerve or plexus can be visualised, there is no specific volume that is recommended. This is dictated by
  - Volume required to surround the nerve [doughnut shaped spread of LA].
  - Volume to stay within the toxic dosage.
- Use adjuvants in children >3 months, or when a longer duration of block is required. Commonly use adjuvants with proven benefit include alpha 2 agonists [clonidine, dexmedetomidine] (Table 6.2).

All the above doses are similar for bupivacaine, levobupivacaine or ropivacaine. However, due to higher safety profile and less motor blockade, levobupivacaine and ropivacaine are the preferred drugs.

Table 6.2 Dosing recommendations [ESRA/ASRA guidelines]

No	Regional block	Dosage
1	Spinal	Neonate-1 mg/kg of Bupivcaine Children > 1 year—0.5 mg/kg of Bupivacaine
2	Caudal	2 mg/kg [maximum dose] Volume is used as per the dermatomal level required
3	Epidural—Bolus	Initial loading dose · Lumbar 0.5 mg/kg · Thoracic 0.3 mg/kg Top ups · 0.25 mg/kg
4	Epidural—infusion	<3 months—0.2 mg/kg/h 3 months–1 year—0.3 mg/kg/h >1 year—0.4 mg/kg/h
5	Limb blocks—single shot	0.5–1.5 mg/kg
6	Fascial plane blocks—single shot	0.25 mg–0.75 mg/kg
7	Limb and fascial plane blocks—continuous infusion	0.1–0.3 mg/kg/h

6.1.6 Complications in Paediatric Regional Anaesthesia

1. Complication rates are higher in children <6 months.
2. Central neuraxial blocks have six times higher complication rate than peripheral nerve block [4].
3. The incidence of complications is not necessarily higher when regional anaesthesia is done under sedation/general anaesthesia, which seems to be the norm in most situations [5].
4. Dosing errors are common. Since paediatrics is a diverse age group, careful consideration should be given to loading drugs after calculating the dosage based on the weight of the child.
5. To minimise complication, more distal blocks [e.g. popliteal approach versus sub gluteal approach to sciatic nerve] are preferred as tourniquet pain is rarely a problem as most also have sedation/general anaesthesia. (Table 6.3).

In this section, we will discuss only regional blocks which are done more commonly or exclusively in paediatrics.

6.2 Head and Neck Blocks

Most blocks done in the head and neck are done using landmark-based techniques. These include scalp nerve blocks, infraorbital, cervical plexus, Arnold nerve block, Greater occipital nerve block. The only block where USG is recommended is for the maxillary nerve block in the pterygopalatine fossa. Greater occipital nerve can also be visualised by USG and is used to improve the success rate.

6.2.1 Maxillary Nerve Block

Anatomy It is a pure sensory branch of the trigeminal nerve supplying the mid part of the face. It leaves the foramen rotundum and enters the pterygopalatine fossa. Its branches are zygomatic nerve, infraorbital nerve, nasopalatine, lesser palatine and greater palatine nerves (Fig. 6.1).

Sonoanatomy The pterygopalatine fossa is located between two bony landmarks—anteriorly maxilla and posteriorly the greater wing of sphenoid.

Technique Suprazygomatic approach, out of plane approach is used. Linear probe is positioned below the zygomatic arch and the needle insertion is above the zygomatic arch at the frontozygomatic angle (Fig. 6.2). The needle is initially advanced perpendicular to the skin to meet the greater wing of the sphenoid. After that it is angled anteriorly [20°] and caudally [10°] into the pterygopalatine fossa. Alternatively, the needle can be angled appropriately into the pterygopalatine fossa through the pterygomaxillary fissure (Fig. 6.2) under USG guidance. A doppler to visualise the internal maxillary artery would prevent injury. The maxillary nerve

Table 6.3 Regional anaesthetic blocks and common surgical indications

Block	Indication
Head and neck	
Scalp block	Craniotomy
Greater occipital nerve block	Posterior craniotomy
Maxillary nerve block	Cleft lip and palate surgery, Septoplasty,
Cervical plexus	Neck—Lymph node biopsy, thyroid surgery, thyroglossal cyst excision, branchial cyst Head—mastoid, tympanic surgery
Auricular branch of Vagus [Arnold nerve]	External auditory canal surgery, myringotomy
Upper limb	
Brachial plexus—Interscalene, supraclavicular, infraclavicular, costoclavicular, axillary	Upper limb procedures
Suprascapular	Shoulder surgery
Individual nerves—Musculocutaneous, median, radial and ulnar	Distal limb procedures, as a rescue block
Lower limb	
Femoral—Classical, adductor canal	Procedure on the femur and knee joint
Lateral femoral cutaneous nerve	Skin graft, muscle biopsy in suspected myopathies
Sciatic—gluteal, popliteal	Knee and procedures distal to it
Truncal anterior	
PECS 1, 2 and Serratus anterior	Anterior chest wall procedures, rib fractures, breast surgery
Pectointercostal fascial plane block Tranversus thoracis muscle plane block	Sternotomy
TAP—classical, subcostal	Laparoscopy and laparotomy
Rectus sheath	Umbilical procedures, midline laparotomy
Ilioinguinal/iliohypogastric	Inguinal hernia, orchidopexy
Truncal posterior	
Erector spinae	Thoracic and abdominal procedures
Quadratus lumborum	Abdominal procedures, Inguinal hernia
Transversalis fascia block	Iliac bone grafting
Paravertebral	CDH repair, thoracotomy, upper abdominal laparotomy, nephrectomy, pyeloplasty
Central neuraxial	1. Spinal 2. Epidural 3. Caudal 4. Trans-sacral [S2–S3]
Perineal	
Dorsal Penile	Penile procedures
Pudendal	Penile, vaginal and perineal procedures

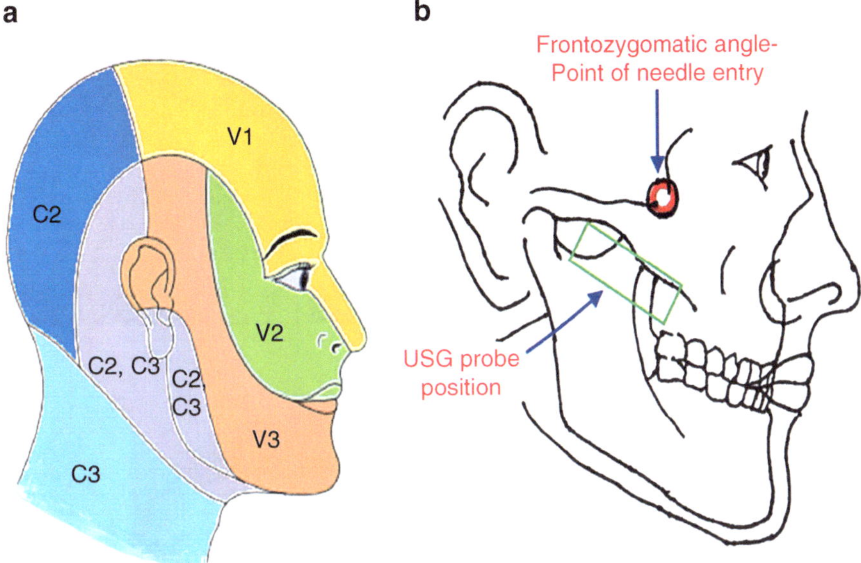

Fig. 6.1 (**a**) Sensory distribution of the maxillary nerve, (**b**) Ultrasound probe position for block

cannot be visualised due to its small size, depth and path parallel to the axis of probe. Once in the fossa, LA can be injected.

6.2.2 Greater Occipital Nerve Block

Used for posterior craniotomies. It is the posterior primary rami from C2 and supplies the posterior part of the neck along with lesser occipital and suboccipital nerve.

Nerve can be identified between two muscles, superiorly—semispinalis capitis and inferiorly—obliquus capitis inferior and it lies medial to the occipital artery.

6.3 Upper Limb Blocks

Approaches to the brachial plexus in the neck are technically more challenging in small children due to the small neck. A head ring and a shoulder roll will create enough room to aid USG probe placement and manoeuvring.

6.4 Truncal Blocks

Most of the truncal blocks are interfascial plane blocks, hence require a larger volume. Due to the thin abdominal wall of infants and small children, it is important that USG is used to perform the injection in the correct site and to avoid intraperitoneal injection or injury to the viscera.

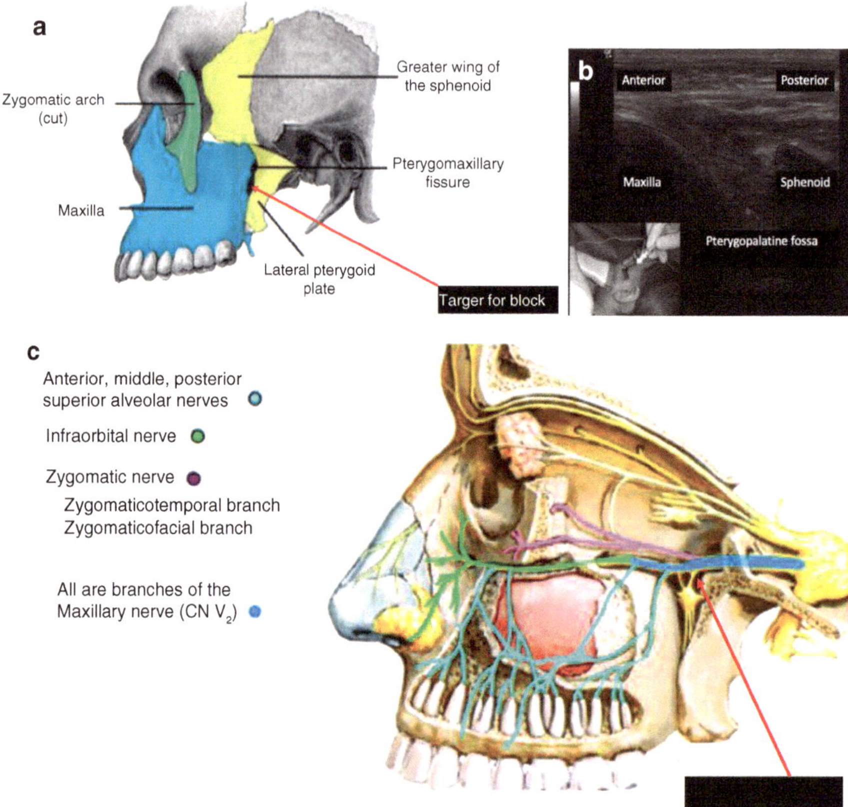

Fig. 6.2 (**a**) Entry to the pterygopalatine fissure, (**b**) Sonoanatomy of pterygopalatine fossa

6.4.1 Thoracic Fascial Plane Blocks (for Details See Chap. 4)

Pectointercostal fascial plane block

The pectointercostal fascial plane block is used for midline incisions over the thorax [e.g. sternotomy].

Plane—LA is deposited between the pectoralis major and the intercostal muscles, 1–2 cm lateral to the lateral border of the sternum with the needle angulated in a lateral to the median direction to avoid injury to the internal thoracic vessels.

It blocks the anterior cutaneous branches of the intercostal nerve.

Tranvsersus Thoracis Muscle Plane Block

It is a deeper version of pectointercostal fascial plane block, where in the LA is deposited between the internal intercostal and transversus thoracis muscle.

PECS 1 and PECS 2

It is used for procedures around the mammary region and anterior minithoracotomy.

PECS 1—LA is injected between pectoralis major and pectoralis minor muscles at the level of third rib. It blocks the medial and lateral pectoral nerves.

PECS 2—LA is injected between P. minor muscle and Serratus anterior at the level of third rib. It blocks the long thoracic nerve, thoracodorsal nerve and lateral cutaneous branches of the intercostal nerves [T2–T6].

SAP [Serratus Anterior Plane Block]

It is used for thoracotomy, rib fractures and other procedures involving the anterolateral chest wall.

The LA is injected above or below the serratus anterior muscle, in the midaxillary line at the level of fifth rib.

It blocks the long thoracic nerve, thoracodorsal nerve and lateral cutaneous branches of IC nerves approximately T2–T9.

6.4.2 Abdominal Fascial Plane Blocks

Inguinal Nerve Blocks

Most commonly used for inguinal herniotomy in children, though due to sparing of the genitofemoral nerve this does not provide complete analgesia for this surgery [6].

These block the ilioinguinal and iliohypogastric nerves.

The LA is injected close to the anterior superior iliac spine, between the internal oblique and transverse abdominis muscle. The iliohypogastric is situated lateral to the ilioinguinal nerve.

TAP block

Used for multiple abdominal procedures, though it provides only somatic analgesia. It is important to be mindful of the maximum dose in four quadrant TAP blocks which might require a considerable volume to be effective.

Rectus Sheath Block

It is used for midline incisions, umbilical hernia repair and port related pain in laparoscopic procedures. The drug is deposited between the rectus muscle and posterior rectus sheath at a dose of 0.1–0.2 ml/kg.

Quadratus Lumborum Block (QLB)

QLB can be considered a posterior extension of the TAP block, though it may provide some visceral analgesia due to the spread of the injectate medially to the paravertebral area.

QLB is used in paediatric abdominal surgeries.

Unilateral surgery like nephrectomies can be provided a continuous QLB catheter for postoperative analgesia.

6.4.3 Erector Spinae Block (ESP)

Erector spinae block in children can be used for perioperative analgesia for thoracic and upper abdominal surgery.

Sacral erector spinae block has been used for perioperative analgesia for anoplasty operation.

6.4.4 Paravertebral Blocks

It is a commonly performed block. Being a deeper block with significant associated complications, it is preferably done by someone who is skilled with the basics of USG guided blocks in small children. The anatomy and techniques are similar to that in adults (Figs. 6.3 and 6.4). Being a relatively superficial structure in infants, space is well seen with a linear probe placed in a horizontal plane, just above the shiny and mobile pleural layer.

6.5 Central Neuraxial Blocks

Neuraxial anaesthesia in children, especially neonates and infants require more precision and dexterity. The target sites are at a depth of less than a centimetre in many blocks. Experience is required and new trainees should always perform these blocks under expert guidance. This is also the age group with the highest risk of persistent

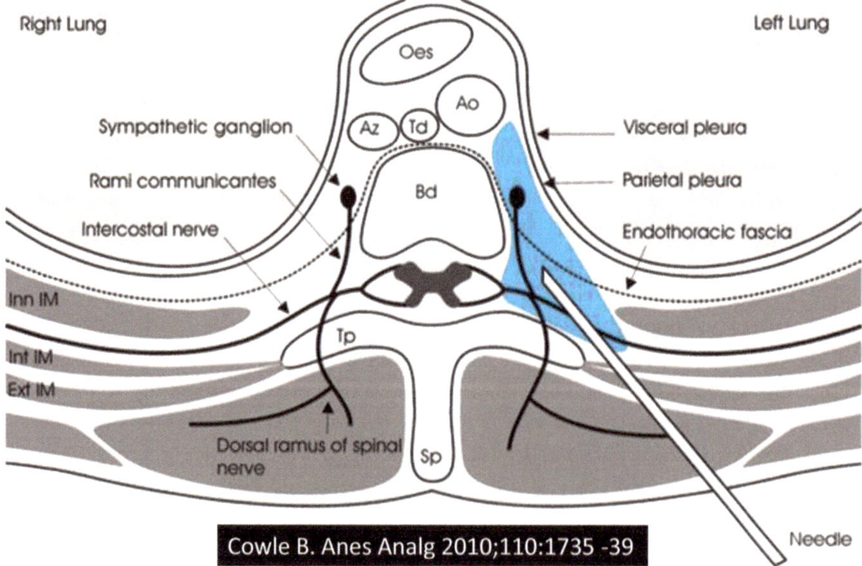

Fig. 6.3 Anatomy of paravertebral space

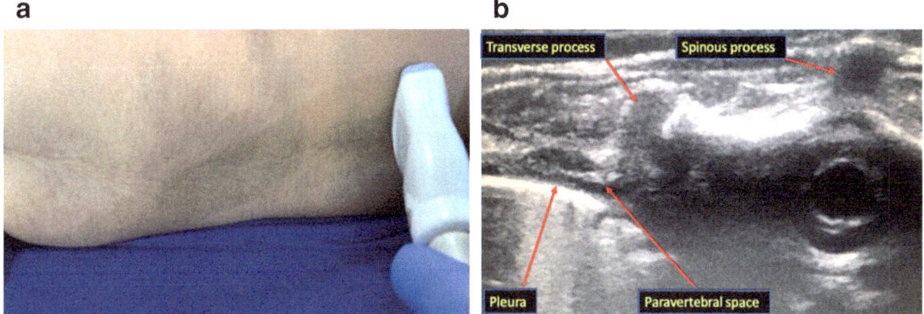

Fig. 6.4 (**a**) Probe position for paravertebral block, (**b**) Sonoanatomy

post-surgical pain and long-term sequelae from inadequately controlled acute pain [7].

6.5.1 Sub-arachnoid Block (SAB)

It is strongly recommended in surgeries for premature born neonates who are less than 50 weeks post-conceptual age to decrease the risk of apnoea. Higher CSF volumes and its turnover mandate a higher dose of LA and result in a shorter duration of action. Spinal is done below the L3 vertebra as the spinal cord ends at this level.

Dose:

- Neonates and small infants—0.5% Bupivacaine 1 mg/kg or 0.2 ml/Kg
- Children > 1 year—0.5% Bupivacaine 0.5 mg/kg or 0.1 ml/kg

6.5.2 Epidural Anaesthesia

Due to incomplete ossification and largely cartilaginous posterior vertebral column, neuraxial structures can be visualised in neonates and small children using USG. Ultrasound can be used to locate the tip of the epidural catheter.

Though ultrasound is still not routinely used for neuraxial blocks, it can be a valuable tool in difficult situations to ascertain

- The point of skin entry
- Assess depth of epidural space
- Detect anatomical abnormalities and variations
- To confirm the tip of the epidural catheter

In neonates, neuraxial structures can be visualised when imaging in the midline sagittal probe position. In other age groups, the images are better with the paramedian sagittal probe position through the interlaminar space.

Various techniques which can be used to locate the tip of the epidural catheter when inserted in the caudal space include

1. Measuring the length from the caudal space to the desired vertebral level and inserting the catheter to the measured length.
2. Styletted epidural catheter can be visualised as a hyperechoic dot in USG.
3. Using electrical stimulation.
4. A small volume of air/saline can be injected through the epidural/caudal catheter.

Epidural catheters can be inserted from the caudal route [8]. However, due to soft ligaments, the risk of dural puncture is high and loss of resistance techniques may not be reliable.

6.5.3 Caudal Anaesthesia

Caudal is the most commonly performed regional anaesthetic block in children. It is preferred over spinal block due to its longer duration, less risk of neural damage and ease of performing the block. Given the fact that the epidural fat is loose and soft, LA injected at the caudal level has the potential to spread to lower thoracic levels. It can provide blockade for all surgeries up to the lower thoracic level.

Caudal can also be used to supplement spinal anaesthesia as the duration of action of subarachnoid block in neonates is shorter compared to older children and adults. In neonates, while doing a caudal, there is a higher risk of dural puncture as the dura ends at S3-4.

Single-shot caudal block/continuous caudal catheter can be used for perioperative analgesia in conjunction with general anaesthesia.

USG is useful over landmark-based caudal in certain situations. These include

1. Obese children.
2. Anatomical variations.
3. Anatomical abnormalities—tuft of hair at the caudal area, nevi over the skin, etc.
4. Failed blind attempt—it is advisable to use the USG if more than three attempts have failed to enter the caudal space.

USG guided caudal has been noted to have a higher success rate at first attempt, with lesser risk of intravascular and subcutaneous injection [9]. USG can also be used to guide the advancement of an epidural catheter placement from the sacral hiatus [10].

Anatomy

Caudal space is generally accessed from the sacral hiatus (Fig. 6.5), which is an inverted U-shaped depression in between two bony prominences at the S4 vertebral level (sacral cornua).

Sonoanatomy

A high-frequency linear ultrasound transducer is used to image the caudal area. Important sonoanatomy landmarks are

- Sacral cornua [bony prominences]: seen as two inverted U-shaped structures.
- Sacrococcygeal ligament—seen as a horizontal hyperechoic line.
- Dorsal surface of sacral bone—seen as a horizontal hyperechoic line beneath the sacrococcygeal ligament.
- Caudal space: Space between the two hyperechoic lines (Fig. 6.6).

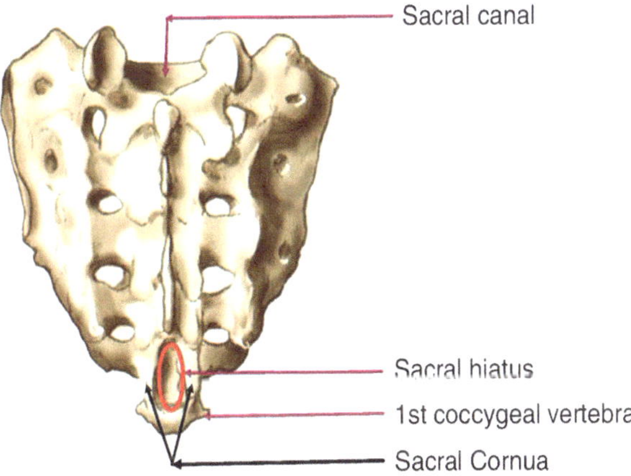

Fig. 6.5 Anatomy of sacral hiatus

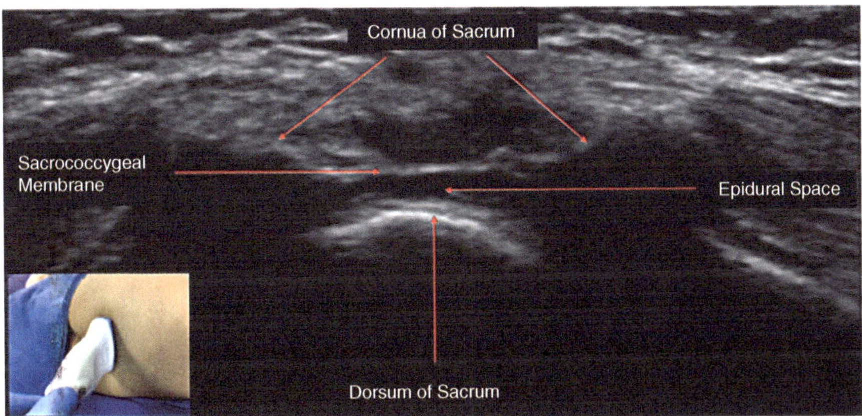

Fig. 6.6 Caudal block: probe position (inset) and sonoanatomy

Technique

After aseptic precautions, the child is made to lie in a lateral or prone position. Caudal space is identified as mentioned above. For single-shot caudal, a spinal needle is used. For inserting the catheter via the caudal route, a short bevel Tuohy needle is inserted out of the plane in a 45° angle from caudal to cephalad direction to access the caudal space. The needle tip can be imaged in the caudal space and test dose of 2–3 ml saline is administered to confirm needle tip location. The spread of the injectate can be imaged by turbulence or Doppler ultrasound.

Alternatively, after locating the caudal space, the probe can be rotated and placed in a sagittal plane in the midline. The block needle can then enter in plane into the caudal space and catheter advancement can be imaged in real time. A small volume (1–2 ml) saline can be injected through the catheter to observe the spread in the epidural space and catheter tip located thus. If the saline spread is difficult to locate, 0.5 ml air can be injected through the catheter to locate its tip.

Note Avoid using hypodermic/hollow needles for caudal or spinal anaesthesia to decrease the risk of epidermoid tumours [implantation dermoid].

6.5.4 Complications of Caudal

These include intravascular, subarachnoid or intrarectal placement of the catheter and local anaesthetic. Urinary retention can be a troublesome side effect. Parents have to warn of potential leg weakness for 4–6 h after a single-shot caudal and to be cautious while mobilising the child.

6.5.5 Trans-sacral Approach to Caudal Space

This is done at the level of S2–3 [11] and USG has shown to have a higher success rate. This technique is an alternative when the identification of sacral hiatus is difficult. Limitation of this approach is the potential puncture of the dura as that the lower end of the dural sac ends at S2.

Recent recommendations suggest peripheral nerve blocks over caudal and spinal, due to a higher risk of complications in central blocks.

6.6 Perineal Blocks

6.6.1 Pudendal Nerve Block

A technique that is increasingly being recommended over caudal due to concerns over potential complications like fistula formation [in hypospadias surgery] and increased risk of bleeding. It also offers a longer duration of sensory block [12], no urinary retention and less risk of motor block. The ventral part of the penis is supplied by the perineal nerve, which is a branch of the pudendal nerve. Hence, it provides a more complete block for penile surgery compared to the dorsal penile nerve block [13]. However, a recent metanalysis suggests that caudal is not associated with a higher risk of complications in hypospadias compared to pudendal or penile nerve blocks [14].

Indications

1. Penile surgery.
2. Vaginal surgery.
3. Anal surgery.
4. Perineal procedures—this may not be possible in transperineal USG guided block as the inferior rectal nerve may not be blocked.

Anatomy

Pudendal nerve arises from the ventral rami of the sacral plexus [S2–4]. It is called the nerve of the perineum as it supplies the perineum and muscles within the perineum, penis, external anal sphincter and posterior 2/3 of scrotum (Fig. 6.7).

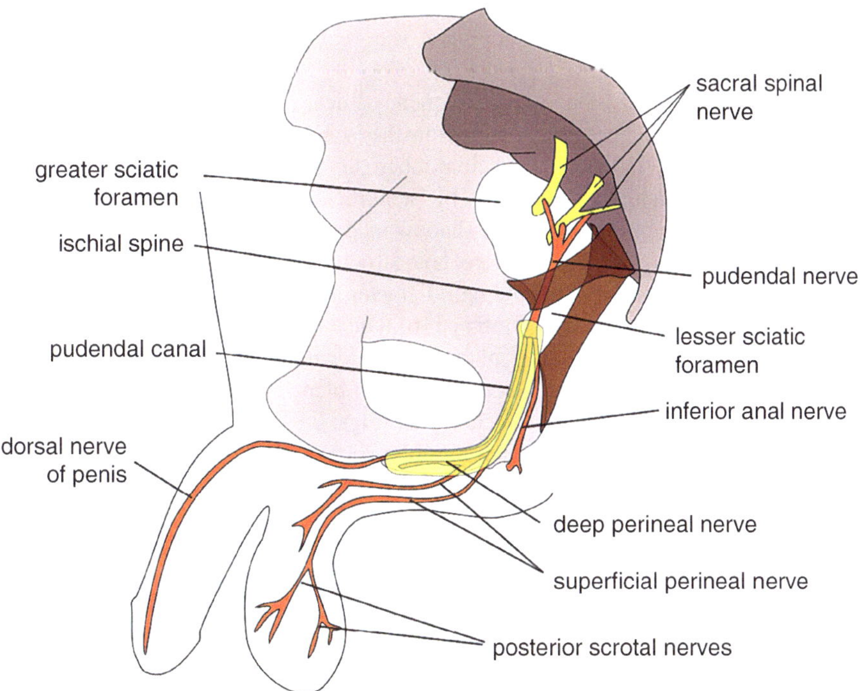

Fig. 6.7 Anatomy of pudendal nerve. Source: *Häggström, Mikael (2014)*. "Medical gallery of Mikael Häggström 2014". *WikiJournal of Medicine 1 (2)*. DOI:https://doi.org/10.15347/wjm/2014.008. ISSN 2002-4436. Public Domain

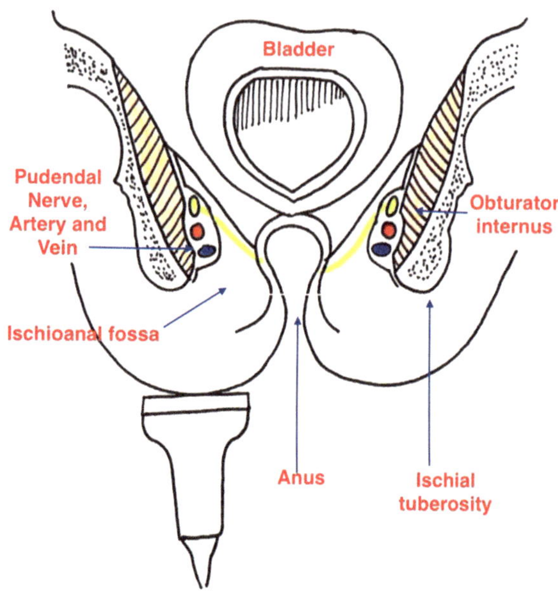

Fig. 6.8 Pudendal nerve block anatomy. (**a**) Transverse and (**b**) oblique parasagittal probe position. Note the needle enters 'out of plane' in (**a**) and 'in plane' in (**b**)

Technique

The ultrasound-guided perineal approach was reported by Parras and Blanco in 2013 [15].

In the lithotomy position, a high-frequency linear probe is placed between the anus and the ischial tuberosity so as to view the ischiorectal fossa. The hyperechoic curved line laterally indicates the ischial tuberosity and the hypoechoic area medially represents the anorectal shadow. The ischiorectal fossa lies between the ischial tuberosity laterally and the anorectal shadow medially. The pudendal nerve may be visualised in the fossa as small hyperechoic structures of about 2 mm. Recognition may be impaired because of their small diameter, and colour Doppler is useful for identifying the internal pudendal artery [16]. Once the vascular structure is identified, the needle is advanced out of plane and the local anesthetic is injected. A dose of 0.5–1 ml/kg on each side is injected. An out of plane approach is used. A dose of 0.4 ml/kg is injected in the ischiorectal fossa (Figs. 6.8 and 6.9).

Alternatively, an oblique parasagittal probe orientation and in plane needling can be used with the needle moving from caudad to cephalad direction.

Limitations of This Block

- Need for a bilateral block [hence the potential for LA toxicity].
- Spread of LA is not well appreciated due to the fat density that makes it almost as anechoic as that of the LA.

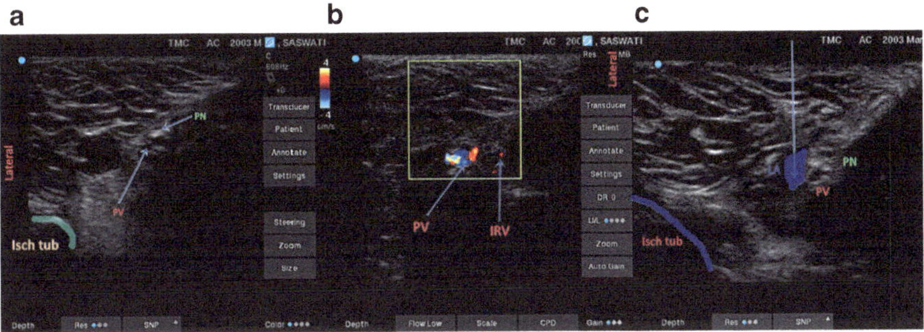

Fig. 6.9 Pudendal nerve block Ultrasound image: (**a**) the initial scanning image, (**b**) Colour Doppler image showing pudendal vessels (PV) and inferior rectal vessels (IRV), (**c**) Pudendal nerve block: the block needle enters out of plane, LA is deposited around the pudendal nerve (PN). Note that the ischial tuberosity (Isch tub) lies lateral and anus/perineal body medial. The above image is of a pudendal nerve block in the right side

- Potential for artery injury, as visualisation of the pudendal artery is difficult due to its small diameter and sinuous path.
- The success rate of 88% [17].

6.6.1.1 Blockmate Pearls

- For better image resolution a 22G × 50 mm echogenic neurostimulation needle can be used.
- Contraction of the anal sphincter confirms that the inferior rectal nerve is close.
- Neurostimulation may not always identify the pudendal nerve [16]; this may be due to the low percentage of motor fibres it contains or the small size of its branches.

6.6.2 Dorsal Penile Nerve Block

Used as an alternative to pudendal or caudal for penile surgery.

Anatomy

The neurovascular bundle in the penis is situated beneath Buck's fascia (deep fascia) on either side of the suspensory ligament of the penis (Figs. 6.10). The structures from medial to lateral are vein, artery and nerve.

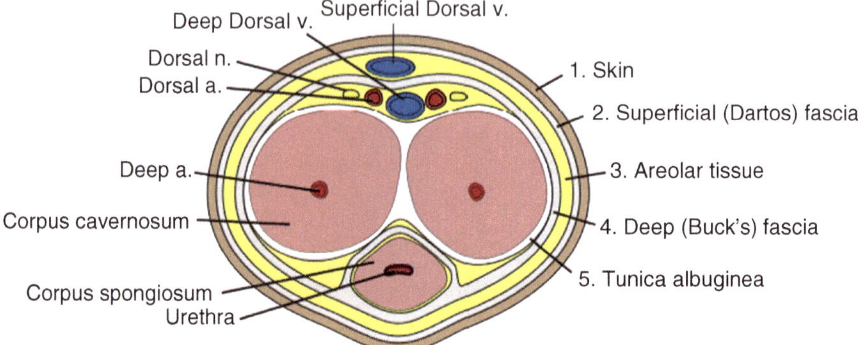

Fig. 6.10 Cross-sectional anatomy of penis. Source: Wikimedia commons. Creative Commons Attribution 3.0 Unported licence

Technique
A high-frequency linear probe is used to image the neurovascular bundle below Buck's fascia. In case the dorsal nerve is not imaged, 2 ml of LA is injected on either side lateral to the artery by piercing the fascia. Additional LA is injected at the peno-scrotal hub to block the scrotal branches of the pudendal nerve which supply the ventral midline skin to the frenulum.

Complications
In the absence of USG there is a potential risk of injury to the nerve, artery or vein.

6.6.2.1 Blockmate Pearls

- Penile arteries are end arteries therefore damage to the artery should be prevented.
- Local anaesthetic mixture should not contain adrenaline for the above-mentioned reason.

Ultrasound guidance offers better safety and efficacy for regional anaesthesia techniques in children. It is important to perform a thorough scan before starting the procedure. The scan helps to locate vital structures such as blood vessels, nerves and viscera in the vicinity and avoid injury to them. While performing any block, knowledge of regional anatomy is essential. Table 6.4 provides a ready reference to the beginner to find the blood vessels while performing USRA and keep them safe.

Table 6.4 Regional anaesthetic blocks and vascular structure in vicinity

Regional anaesthetic	Artery
Rectus sheath	Superior epigastric Artery [above umbilicus] Inferior epigastric artery [below umbilicus]
Supraclavicular nerve block	Subclavian artery lies inferomedial to plexus Transverse cervical artery can be seen
PECS 1 block	Thoracoacromial artery lies between the P. Major and P. Minor
Inguinal nerve block	Deep circumflex iliac artery lies medial to the two nerves
Occipital nerve block	Occipital artery lies lateral to it
Median nerve at elbow	Brachial artery lies medial to it
Infraclavicular block	Three cords seen around the axillary artery Medial cord at 3 o'clock position Posterior cord—6 o'clock position Lateral cord—9 o'clock position
Forearm level—ulnar nerve	Ulnar artery runs lateral to it
Forearm level—radial nerve	Radial artery runs medial to it
Femoral nerve	Femoral artery is medial to it
Popliteal Fossa—sciatic nerve	Popliteal artery is superolateral to it
Pudendal nerve block	Pudendal artery
Pectointercostal nerve block	Internal thoracic artery

References

1. Suresh S, Ecoffey C, Bosenberg A, Lonnqvist PA, De Oliveira GS, de Leon Casasola O, De Andrés J, Ivani G. The European Society of Regional Anaesthesia and Pain Therapy/American Society of Regional Anesthesia and Pain Medicine recommendations on local anesthetics and adjuvants dosage in pediatric regional anesthesia. Reg Anesth Pain Med. 2018 Feb 1;43(2):211–6.
2. Walker BJ, Long JB, Sathyamoorthy M, et al. Complications in pediatric regional anesthesia: an analysis of more than 100,000 blocks from the Pediatric Regional Anesthesia Network. Anesthesiology. 2018;129:721–32.
3. Dadure C, Veyckemans F, Bringuier S, Habre W. Epidemiology of regional anesthesia in children: lessons learned from the European Multi-Institutional Study APRICOT. Paediatr Anaesth. 2019;29:1128–35.
4. Giaufre E, Dalens B, Gombert A. Epidemiology and morbidity of regional anesthesia in children: a one-year prospective survey of the French-Language Society of Pediatric Anesthesiologists. Anesth Analg. 1996;83:904–12.
5. Ecoffey C, Lacroix F, Giaufre E, et al. Epidemiology and morbidity of regional anesthesia in children: a follow-up one year prospective survey of the French-Language Society of Pediatric Anaesthesiologists. Pediatr Anesth. 2010;20:1061–9.
6. Willschke H, Kettner S. Pediatric regional anesthesia: abdominal wall blocks. Pediatr Anesth. 2012;22:82–92.
7. Taddio A, Katz J, Ilersich AL, Koren G. Effect of neonatal circumcision on pain response during subsequent routine vaccination. Lancet. 1997;349:599–603.
8. Willschke H, Bosenberg A, Marhofer P, Willschke J, Schwindt J, Weintraud M, et al. Epidural catheter placement in neonates: sonoanatomy and feasibility of ultrasonographic guidance in term and preterm neonates. Reg Anesth Pain Med. 2007;32:34–40.

9. Ahiskalioglu A, Yayik AM, Ahiskalioglu EO, Ekinci M, Gölboyu BE, Celik EC, et al. Ultrasound-guided versus conventional injection for caudal block in children: a prospective randomized clinical study. J Clin Anesth. 2018;44:91–6.
10. Ponde VC, Bedekar VV, Desai AP, Puranik KA. Does ultrasound guidance add accuracy to continuous caudal-epidural catheter placements in neonates and infants? Paediatr Anaesth. 2017;27:1010–4.
11. Busoni P, Sarti A. Sacral intervertebral epidural block. Anesthesiology. 1987;67:993–5.
12. Naja ZM, Ziade FM, Kamel R, El-Kayali S, Daoud N, El-Rajab MA. The effectiveness of pudendal nerve block versus caudal block anesthesia for hypospadias in children. Anesth Analg. 2013;117:1401–7.
13. Kendigelen P, Tutuncu AC, Emre S, Altindas F, Kaya G. Pudendal versus caudal block in children undergoing hypospadias surgery: a randomized controlled trial. Reg Anesth Pain Med. 2016;41:610–5.
14. Zhu C, Wei R, Tong Y, Liu J, Song Z, Zhang S. Analgesic efficacy and impact of caudal block on surgical complications of hypospadias repair: a systematic review and meta-analysis. Reg Anesth Pain Med. 2019 Feb 1;44(2):259–67.
15. Parras T, Blanco R. Bloqueo pudendo ecoguiado/Ultrasond guided pudendal block. Cir Mayor Ambul. 2013;18:31–5.
16. Rofaeel A, Peng P, Louis I, Chan V. Feasibility of real-time ultrasound for pudendal nerve block in patients with chronic perineal pain. Reg Anesth Pain Med. 2008;33:139–45.
17. Gaudet-Ferrand I, De La Arena P, Bringuier S, Raux O, Hertz L, Kalfa N, Sola C, Dadure C. Ultrasound-guided pudendal nerve block in children: a new technique of ultrasound-guided transperineal approach. Pediat Anesth. 2018 Jan;28(1):53–8.

Recent Advances in Regional Anaesthesia

7

Chang Chuan Melvin Lee, Arunangshu Chakraborty, and Shri Vidya

7.1 Introduction

The practice of regional anaesthesia has evolved significantly over the past decade. We have seen a transition from anatomical landmark-based techniques with or without nerve stimulator-guidance, to ultrasound guidance as a new standard-of-care in most developed healthcare systems [1, 2]. The introduction of ultrasonography—which has become more advanced and accessible, has revolutionised the practice of regional anaesthesia, set a new standard-of-care [1, 2], and improved competency in core techniques for the average anaesthetic provider. Ultrasound-guided regional anaesthesia also allows for improved success rates, may decrease complications [3], as well as facilitate novel approaches to peripheral nerve blockade, such as fascial plane blocks. The practice of regional anaesthesia has also since evolved from being a simple alternative to general anaesthesia. With increasing recognition of the deleterious effects of opioid-based anaesthesia and pain management, regional anaesthesia is increasingly viewed as part of a multimodal anaesthetic and pain management strategy.

7.2 Expanding Roles

Regional anaesthesia is increasingly being viewed as more than just an alternative to general anaesthesia. Regional anaesthesia blunts the stress response to surgery, and reduces, or even avoids exposure to central nervous system depressants and

C. C. M. Lee (✉)
National University Health System, Singapore, Singapore

A. Chakraborty
Department of Anaesthesia, CC and Pain, Tata Medical Center, Kolkata, India

S. Vidya
Anaesthesiology, National University Health System, Singapore, Singapore

A. Chakraborty (ed.), *Blockmate*, https://doi.org/10.1007/978-981-15-9202-7_7

opioids. In total hip and knee arthroplasty, neuraxial anaesthesia has been associated with a reduction in patient mortality, major morbidity (e.g. pulmonary complications, transfusion requirements) and economic outcomes such as length of hospital stay when compared to general anaesthesia [4, 5]. This has seen an increasing interest in recent years, with the emergence of fast-tracking and enhanced recovery from surgery. Effective post-operative analgesia with less reliance on opioid-based analgesic regimens can reduce ileus, allow early mobilisation, physical therapy, and hasten recovery and discharge from hospital [6, 7]. The reduction in sedative and systemic opioid burden by regional anaesthesia—either as a sole technique or adjunct to general anaesthesia may, theoretically, have benefits on delirium and post-operative cognitive dysfunction; particularly with an increasing number of elderly presenting for surgical procedures. However, this is yet to be conclusively demonstrated, likely due to the complex physiological changes in the perioperative period of which anaesthesia is just one facet of [8, 9]. Regional anaesthesia may also have benefits which extend into surgical outcomes—vasodilation from sympatholysis due to regional anaesthesia has been purported to improve patency rate and success in arteriovenous fistula creation surgery [10, 11]. Regional anaesthesia has also been advocated in oncological surgery to reduce the risk of cancer recurrence. Purported benefits include effective suppression of the surgical inflammatory response, preservation of immune function, a direct action of systemic local anaesthetics (LA) on tumour cell apoptosis, and indirectly through reduction in the use of opioids which may promote metastasis [12–15].

7.3 Technological Advances

Ultrasound guidance has contributed to the efficacy and safety of regional anaesthesia provision, compared to neurostimulation alone. Visualisation of underlying structures allows for identification of anatomical variants, avoids accidental vascular puncture, and allows for peripheral nerve blockade to be performed with reductions in minimum local anaesthetic dose requirements [3, 16]. This translates into a reduced risk of local anaesthetic systemic toxicity, although a similar benefit in reducing neurological complications has yet to be conclusively demonstrated [17, 18]—likely due to the low event rate [16, 19] and multifactorial aetiology of neurological injury in the perioperative period.

Needle tip identification is crucial when performing ultrasound-guided regional anaesthesia. Challenges to accurate, consistent needle tip visualisation include the proper alignment of the needle (for in-plane approaches) to the ultrasound beam, artefacts, and steep insertion angles which result in poor specular reflection. The best needle visualisation occurs when the angle of incidence is zero, which maximises reflected ultrasound waves; however, at steeper insertion angles, reflection of ultrasound waves away from the transducer degrades image quality. Technical advances have led to improved needle visualisation under ultrasonographic guidance by addressing these issues. While physical probe-mounted needle guides

(CIVCO Medical Solutions, Iowa, United States of America) have been employed previously as an aid for the novice operator to improve needle alignment, the advent of textured echogenic needles (e.g. Stimuplex® Ultra 360®, BBraun Melsungen AG, Melsungen, Germany and SonoPlex®, Pajunk GmbH, Geisingen, Germany) (Figs. 7.1 and 7.2) has been increasingly adopted and have further improved comfort and competence in needle placement and manipulation under ultrasound [20–23]. Such needles are textured with embossed structures along the needle surface, such as cornerstone reflections (SonoPlex®, Pajunk GmbH, Geisingen, Germany) which increase direct and indirect reflection of ultrasound waves back to the probe, even at steep insertion angles [20, 21].

Emerging developments in needle-guidance technology have the potential to improve success rates and increase the safety of ultrasound-guided regional anaesthesia by facilitating needle-beam alignment [22, 23]. Systems employing electromagnetic tracking (eTRAX, Civco, and SonixGPS®, UltraSonix, Richmond, BC, Canada), camera tracking, fibre-optic hydrophones, and tip-mounted sensors have all been described [24–27]. A needle with a piezoelectric sensor mounted close to

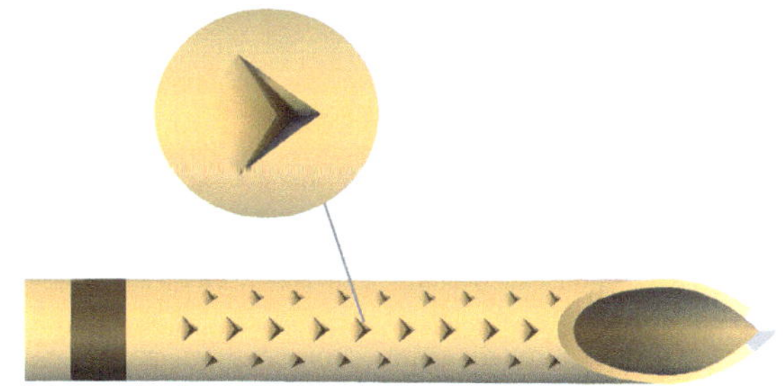

Fig. 7.1 Cornerstone reflectors: the reflectors are engravings on the needle surface designed to improve reflection of ultrasound beams at any angle

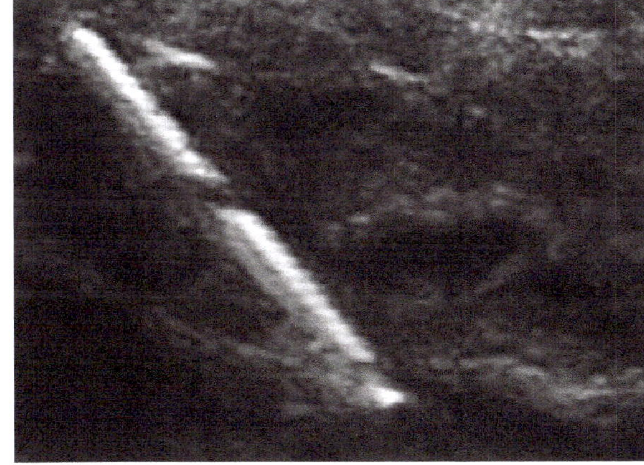

Fig. 7.2 Cornerstone reflectors along the needle surface of an echogenic needle (Pajunk®) designed to improve reflection of ultrasound waves, thus improving needle visualisation, even at steep insertion angels. The distal portion of the needle comprises two echogenic segments 10 mm each (Reproduced with permission, Pajunk® GmbH, Geisingen, Germany)

the needle tip (StimuplexOnvision®, B Braun Melsungen AG, Melsungen, Germany) (Fig. 7.3) has been recently launched. Linked to an ultrasound console (Xperius®, Philips Medical Systems International BV, Eindhoven, The Netherlands), the sensor transfers information to a signal processing unit which calculates and projects, via an image processing unit, the needle tip position, onto the two-dimensional (2D) image as a circle. Multiplanar three-dimensional (3D) and four-dimensional (4D) ultrasound imaging have the potential to better delineate anatomy, improve spatial orientation, and offer real-time assessment of needle positioning and spread of injected local anaesthetic [23, 24]. Additionally, advanced imaging modalities such as elastography may be applied to regional anesthesia to differentiate neural structures from surrounding tissue. Strain elastography is a qualitative technique which provides an indirect measure of tissue stiffness in

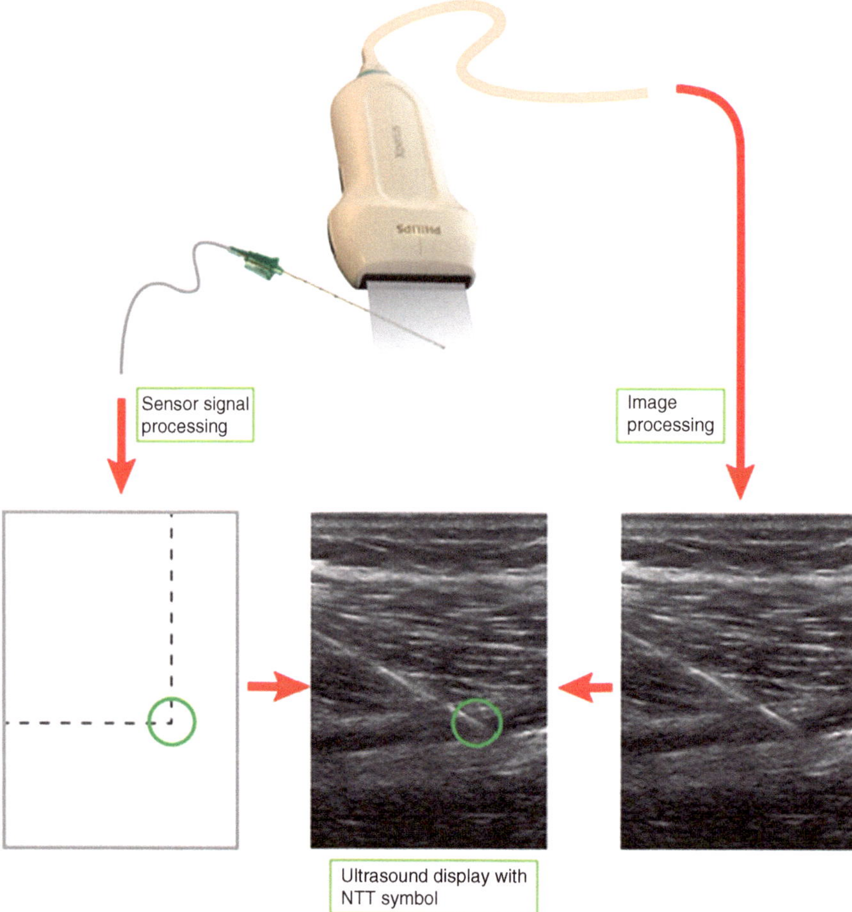

Fig. 7.3 The StimuplexOnvision® (B Braun Melsungen AG, Melsungen, Germany) (From: Kåsine, T, Romundstad, L, Rosseland, LA, et al. Needle tip tracking for ultrasound-guided peripheral nerve block procedures—An observer blinded, randomised, controlled, crossover study on a phantom model. *Acta Anaesthesiol Scand*. 2019; 63: 1055–1062. https://doi.org/10.1111/aas.13379)

response to an applied force - and can potentially be used to assess the spread of local anaesthetic from changes in tissue elasticity. Shear wave elastography allows for qualitative and quantitative measurement of tissue elasticity, by tracking the resultant shear waves propagated from tissue displacement by ultrasonography, termed acoustic radiation force imaging (ARFI). Shear wave elastography may see potential in differentiating needle and nerves from surrounding tissues by generation of a colorized map of differing tissue stiffness [20, 28]. Such advances, which are not yet employed in regional anaesthesia, may be potential methods of improving success and safety of regional anaesthesia in the years to come.

7.4 Injection Pressure Monitoring

Whilst ultrasound has improved the safety and efficacy of regional anaesthesia, it has limitations despite its popularity. Apart from being operator-dependent, deep structures are less well visualised, making identification of a sonographic target difficult, and appreciation of needle-nerve proximity even more so. In such cases, neurostimulation can help locate neural structures with poor sonographic imaging. However, this too is limited by poor specificity in identifying needle-nerve proximity, as well as unreliable once LA injection has commenced; thus potentially increasing the risk of inadvertent nerve injury, particularly with multi-injection techniques. A 2015 consensus statement from the American Society of Regional Anaesthesia and Pain Medicine has expanded the recommendations to include injection pressure monitoring for earlier detection of needle-nerve contact and consequent intrafascicular injection of LA [29]. An opening pressure in excess of 15 psi has been recommended as suggestive of needle-nerve contact (Gadsden et al. 2014) [30, 31]. Commercial kits for monitoring of injection pressure are available, and improvised techniques, such as a half-the-air technique using a central three-way stopcock with a test syringe containing normal saline or 5% dextrose for pressure monitoring and hydrolocation (Lin and Lu 2014) [32] (Fig. 7.4). An alternative approach adopted

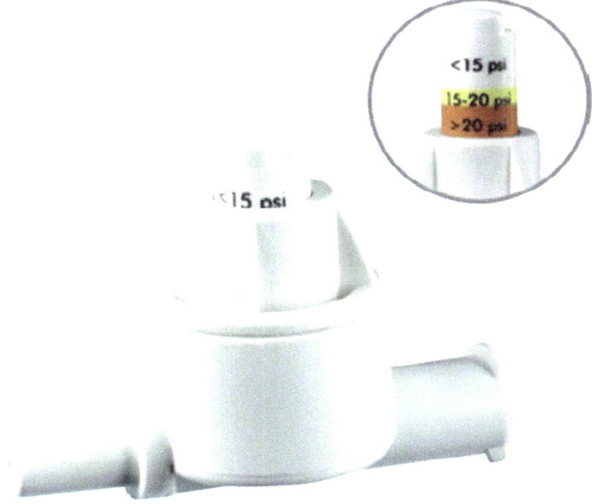

Fig. 7.4 A commercially available, disposable in-line injection pressure monitoring device (Reproduced with permission, BBraun Melsungen AG, Melsungen, Germany)

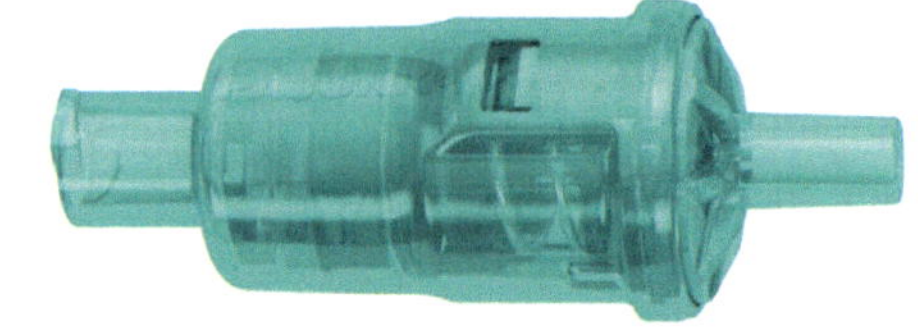

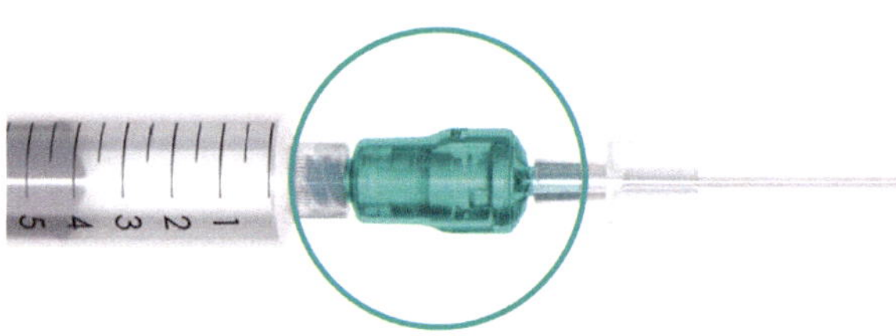

Fig. 7.5 An injection pressure limiting device, which prevents injection when the opening pressure exceeds 15 psi (Reproduced with permission, NerveGuard™, Pajunk GmbH, Geisingen, Germany)

has been to utilise an injection pressure limiter (NerveGuard™, Pajunk GmbH, Geisingen, Germany) (Fig. 7.5) to prevent injection if the opening pressure exceeds 15 psi, thus theoretically allowing identification of an inappropriate needle position, and reducing injections performed with excessive pressure.

7.5 Novel Approaches to Regional Anaesthesia

The introduction of ultrasound in regional anaesthesia has allowed the introduction of new techniques, in addition to improving the efficacy of previously described approaches. Regional anaesthesia techniques that involve an injection of local anaesthetic into fascial planes rather than directly around discrete nerves have seen a rise in popularity due to their ease of performance and safety profiles, making them attractive alternatives to thoracic epidural and paravertebral blockade for truncal analgesia in thoracic and abdominal surgical procedures. These include the Pecs 1 and 2, quadratus lumborum, serratus anterior plane, and erector spinae plane blocks [33–39]. The latter has been described in providing post-operative analgesia in cardiac surgery - particularly minimally-invasive cardiac surgical procedures via a thoracotomy incision, and may be more attractive compared to a thoracic epidural block, as it potentially circumvents the problems associated with an inadvertent vascular puncture in the context of systemic heparinization for cardio-pulmonary bypass [39]. The use of ultrasound has also allowed the blockade of pure sensory nerves otherwise unidentifiable by nerve stimulation alone, such as the adductor canal block which can be employed to provide analgesia following knee arthroplasty [40]. Lastly, the application of ultrasonography has allowed for novel approaches to be established techniques, such as spinal anaesthesia. Ultrasonography is increasingly employed to identify anatomical landmarks in challenging patients, such as the spinous processes delineating the midline, and the depth of the epidural space. Additionally, novel approaches, such as a real-time ultrasound-guided paramedian spinal (Conroy et al. 2013) have been described [41].

7.6 Closed-Loop Systems

A proportion of patients may require sedation when performing regional anaesthesia, and the presence of an experienced, trained anaesthetic provider is an important determinant of patient safety [42, 43]. Administration of anaesthesia and sedation requires continual assessment of the patient's physiological state using monitors and clinical observation. However, as with all procedures, the conduct of regional anaesthesia, especially in cases with challenging anatomy, may prove to be a distraction from patient care. Closed-loop control of sedation and monitoring may be a potential tool that can be implemented to enhance patient safety. Although using monitors supplements clinical observation of the patient, it is nonetheless, by no means a substitute for vigilance and careful observation. However, automated, computerised methods of patient monitoring may be coupled with closed-loop control systems, have been proposed [42–45] and may have the advantage of saving and analysing trends over a time period. Such systems can utilise sensors such as capnography and chest wall impedance to detect apnoeic episodes in addition to standard intraoperative monitors; other potential sensors include processed electroencephalography systems such as the Bispectral index to detect oversedation, accelerometers to detect movement, or image-recognition technologies to detect changes in facial expression. When coupled to systems that process this information and mimic human decision processes—this potential to titrate sedation frees the human operator to focus on the procedure or on other aspects of anaesthetic care provision and acts as an additional safety net.

7.7 Pharmacological Agents

Prolongation of the analgesic effect provided by local anaesthetics is attractive to cover the duration of acute post-operative pain, facilitate recovery, and provide patient comfort and satisfaction that extends well into the post-operative period. However, the action of most commercially available local anaesthetic preparations do not extend beyond 18–24 h, and beyond that, catheter-based techniques are generally required. Catheter-based techniques harbour multiple problems—they require appropriate expertise to place, are susceptible to tip migration (and dislodgement), are at risk of being blocked or kinked, shearing, block failure, nerve irritation, local inflammation and infection; in addition, they may require specialised delivery systems for local anaesthetic delivery.

7.8 Novel Formulations

Novel formulations providing sustained-release of local anaesthetic are attractive, although encapsulating agents such as liposomes and microspheres are required to prevent systemic absorption and systemic toxicity for a large dose of injected local anaesthetic. Liposomes consist of a lipid bilayer with an internal aqueous space in which hydrophilic drugs such as local anaesthetics can be encapsulated, slowing the release rate of local anaesthetics such as Bupivacaine [46–48]. However, their use is limited by a difficult, expensive manufacturing process; and concerns regarding uncontrolled leakage of local anaesthetic as well as neurotoxicity of the encapsulating agent still remain. More importantly, conclusive evidence that there is any meaningful improvement in analgesia, or reduction in opioid use or adverse events has yet to be demonstrated [46, 47, 49].

7.9 Adjuncts

The addition of different agents to the local anaesthetic mixture has been described in regional anaesthesia, and several proven to be effective in prolonging the duration of analgesia without motor blockade [2].

The ideal adjuvant should preferably display the characteristic features:

1. Improve the quality of sensory blockade
2. Prolong the duration of sensory blockade
3. Preferentially affect sensory blockade over motor blockade
4. Shorten the speed of onset of the LA
5. Reduce the LA dosage required
6. No local irritant effects
7. Low allergenic potential
8. High therapeutic index
9. Not neurotoxic; should not increase the risk of adverse neurological outcomes
10. Have minimal systemic absorption and adverse effects
11. Cost-effective and readily available

Although no one agent exists with all the features, many have been identified for its use as an adjunct. As with all medications and procedures, a careful assessment of the risk-benefit ratio must be undertaken prior to addition of an adjuvant into the injectate. Recent advances in new drug development, as well as studies of existing agents—such as Dexamethasone [2, 50, 51], have further increased the repertoire of agents available. Notably, the availability of Dexmedetomidine, a α2-adrenoceptor agonist widely employed as a sedative in intensive care units, has been described as an adjuvant in regional anaesthesia. Dexmedetomidine has an eightfold greater specificity for the α2-adrenoceptor compared to its predecessor, Clonidine, which has been shown in multiple studies to be effective in prolonging block duration [52–54]. Clonidine prolongs the sensory blockade of short and medium acting LAs to 2–3 h, and that of long-acting LAs to up to 10 h. The effect of Clonidine is postulated to be due to decreased excitability of neuronal transmission of nociceptive C fibres by increasing the expression of inhibitory K channels. In addition, α1-mediated tissue vasoconstriction decreases the absorption of the injectate. Clonidine also has anti-inflammatory effects—which have also been described with Dexmedetomidine. Dexmedetomidine as an adjuvant in a LA injectate hastens the mean time to onset of sensory blockade by 9 min and that of motor blockade by 8 min; it also prolongs the mean duration of analgesia by approximately 4.5 h (sensory blockade by 4 h and motor blockade by 3.5 h). Dexmedetomidine is also purported to have neuroprotective effects by inhibition of activated nuclear factor NF-κB. However, systemic effects as a result of absorption of any adjuvant has to be considered, and Dexmedetomidine has the potential to produce sedation, bradycardia, and hypotension when given systemically.

7.10 Advances in Catheter Design

Clearly, the use of novel LA formulations and adjuncts can only result in a prolongation of the sensory blockade into the early post-operative period, beyond which catheter-based techniques are still the most practical means of extending analgesia with regional techniques. For decades, the most commonly employed delivery system for perineural catheter placement employed catheters that are inserted either through or over a straight hollow-bore needle. Catheter-through-needle designs have the potential for infusate leak, as a needle is used to penetrate the skin, and a tubing with a smaller diameter fed through the needle—the skin defect is thus a larger hole with a smaller catheter exiting it, allow leakage of fluid at the insertion site—reported to be between 3 and 30% [55]. However, the development of catheter-over-needle devices, akin to the intravenous cannula, allows for less leak (Edwards et al. 2018) as the largest defect is now created by the catheter itself, allowing for a snug fit and ability to withstand higher injectate pressures [55]. Subsequently, in 2018, the US Food and Drug Administration approved the introduction of suture-style catheters, comprising of a catheter with echogenic markings

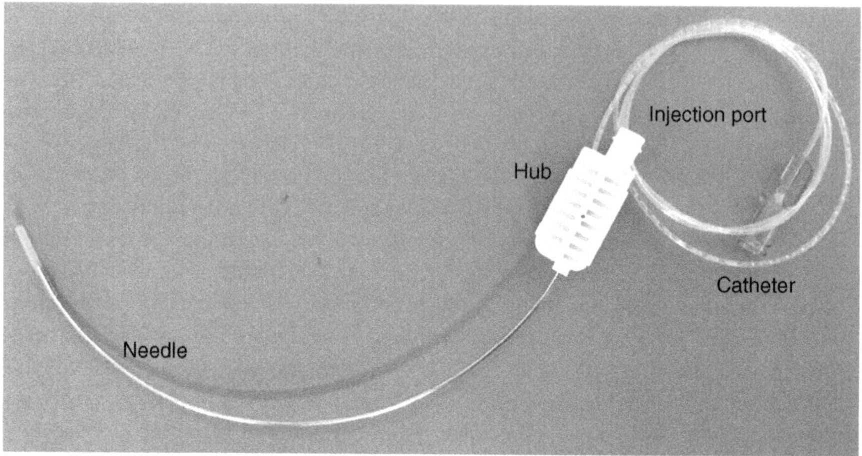

Fig. 7.6 The suture-method catheter (From: Jordahn, Z.M., Lyngeraa, T.S., Grevstad, U. et al. Ultrasound-guided repositioning of a new suture-method catheter for adductor canal block—a randomized pilot study in healthy volunteers. *BMC Anesthesiol* 18, 150 (2018). https://doi.org/10.1186/s12871-018-0615-4)

attached to a hollow, suture-shaped needle (Certa Catheter™; Ferrosan Medical Devices, Szczecin, Poland). (Figs 7.6 and 7.7) The needle can be inserted under ultrasound guidance, through the skin and placed adjacent to the target nerve, pulling the catheter through tissue; the needle is then directed through a separate exit site [56, 57]. The needle can then be disengaged from the catheter, and the catheter secured at both entry and exit sites—thus potentially reducing the risk of dislodgement. This also allows for more precise placement of the catheter compared to catheter-through-needle and catheter-over-needle techniques which 'blindly' advance the catheter past a needle tip positioned adjacent to the nerve.

7.11 Machine Learning and Image Recognition

Lastly, as many medical and non-medical fields begin to incorporate machine-learning in various capacities, it would be unsurprising if ultrasound-guided regional anaesthesia would see image-recognition technology being gradually introduced, as nerve identification can be considered of the more challenging tasks for the novice regional anaesthesia provider. However, compared to other high-fidelity imaging modalities such as computerised tomography and magnetic resonance imaging,

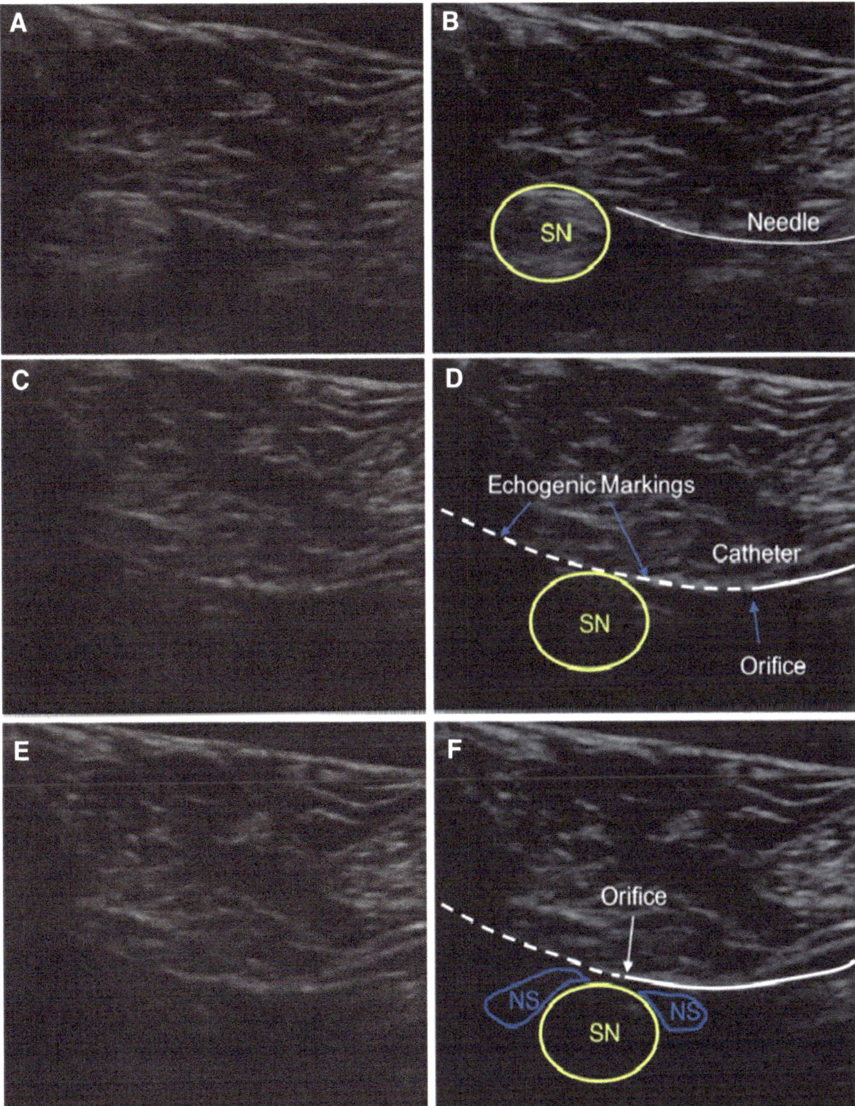

Fig. 7.7 Ultrasound placement of a suture-method catheter. The echogenic markings on the catheter are used to position the orifice adjacent to the nerve. The orifice is located where the echogenic markings terminate. *NS* normal saline, *SN* sciatic nerve (From: Finneran JJ 4th, Gabriel RA, Swisher MW, et al. Suture Catheter for Rescue Perineural Catheter Placement When Unable to Position a Conventional Through-the-Needle Catheter: A Case Report. *A Pract.* 2019;13(9):338–341. doi:10.1213/XAA.0000000000001075)

ultrasonography poses inherent challenges of operator-dependence, and noise and artifacts which degrade image quality. Nonetheless, deep learning has been successfully applied to medical ultrasound imaging tasks such as image classification, object detection, as well as segmentation [58]. Notably, automated software has been deployed in other ultrasound applications [59] such as detection and segmentation of endocardial structures to calculate indices of myocardial function in commercially available platforms (HeartModel[A.I.], Philips Healthcare) [60, 61], and a machine-learning model has been employed in ultrasound images of the femoral nerve and brachial plexus (Huang et al. 2019; Smistad et al. 2018) [62, 63] which further substantiates its viability for exciting future applications in clinical use, and in regional anaesthesia training [64].

References

1. Sen S, Ge M, Prabhakar A, et al. Recent technological advancements in regional anesthesia. Best Pract Res Clin Anaesthesiol. 2019;33(4):499–505. https://doi.org/10.1016/j.bpa.2019.07.002.
2. Albrecht E, Chin KJ. Advances in regional anaesthesia and acute pain management: a narrative review. Anaesthesia. 2020;75:e101–10. https://doi.org/10.1111/anae.14868.
3. Admir Hadzic, Xavier Sala-Blanch, Daquan Xu. Ultrasound Guidance May Reduce but Not Eliminate Complications of Peripheral Nerve Blocks. Anesthesiology. 2008:108(4):557–58.
4. Memtsoudis SG, Sun X, Chiu YL, et al. Perioperative comparative effectiveness of anesthetic technique in orthopedic patients. Anesthesiology. 2013;118:1046–58.
5. Perlas A, Chan VW, Beattie S. Anesthesia technique and mortality after total Hip or Knee Arthroplasty: a retrospective. Propensity Score-matched Cohort Study. Anesthesiology. 2016;125:724–31.
6. McIsaac DI, Cole ET, McCartney CJ. Impact of including regional anaesthesia in enhanced recovery protocols: a scoping review. Br J Anaesth. 2015;115(Suppl 2):ii46–56. https://doi.org/10.1093/bja/aev376.
7. Helander EM, Webb MP, Bias M, Whang EE, Kaye AD, Urman RD. Use of regional anesthesia techniques: analysis of institutional enhanced recovery after surgery protocols for colorectal surgery. J Laparoendosc Adv Surg Tech A. 2017;27(9):898–902. https://doi.org/10.1089/lap.2017.0339.
8. Davis N, Lee M, Lin AY, et al. Postoperative cognitive function following general versus regional anesthesia: a systematic review. J Neurosurg Anesthesiol. 2014;26(4):369–76. https://doi.org/10.1097/ANA.0000000000000120.
9. Mason SE, Noel-Storr A, Ritchie CW. The impact of general and regional anesthesia on the incidence of post-operative cognitive dysfunction and post-operative delirium: a systematic review with meta-analysis. J Alzheimers Dis. 2010;22(Suppl 3):67–79. https://doi.org/10.3233/JAD-2010-101086.
10. Cerneviciute R, Sahebally SM, Ahmed K, et al. Regional versus local anaesthesia for haemodialysis arteriovenous fistula formation: a systematic review and meta-analysis. Eur J Vasc Endovasc Surg. 2017;53:734–42.
11. Armstrong RA, Wilson C, Elliott L, et al. Regional anaesthesia practice for arteriovenous fistula formation surgery. Anaesthesia. 2020;75(5):626–33. https://doi.org/10.1111/anae.14983.
12. Sessler DI, Pei L, Huang Y, et al. Recurrence of breast cancer after regional or general anaesthesia: a randomised controlled trial. Lancet. 2019;394(10211):1807–15. https://doi.org/10.1016/S0140-6736(19)32313-X.
13. Tedore T. Regional anaesthesia and analgesia: relationship to cancer recurrence and survival. Br J Anaesth. 2015;115(Suppl 2):ii34–45. https://doi.org/10.1093/bja/aev375.

14. Cata JP. Outcomes of regional anesthesia in cancer patients. Curr Opin Anaesthesiol. 2018;31:593–600.
15. Divatia JV, Ambulkar R. Anesthesia and cancer recurrence: what is the evidence? J Anaesthesiol Clin Pharmacol. 2014;30(2):147–50. https://doi.org/10.4103/0970-9185.129990.
16. Marhofer P, Harrop-Griffiths W, Willschke H, Kirchmair L. Fifteen years of ultrasound guidance in regional anaesthesia: Part 2-recent developments in block techniques. Br J Anaesth. 2010;104(6):673–83. https://doi.org/10.1093/bja/aeq086. Epub 2010 Apr 23.
17. Marhofer P, Greher M, Kapral S. Ultrasound guidance in regional anaesthesia. Br J Anaesth. 2005;94(1):7–17. https://doi.org/10.1093/bja/aei002.
18. Hebl JR. Ultrasound-guided regional anesthesia and the prevention of neurologic injury: fact or fiction? Anesthesiology. 2008;108(2):186–8. https://doi.org/10.1097/01.anes.0000299835.04104.02.
19. Yves Auroy, Dan Benhamou, Laurent Bargues, Claude Ecoffey, Bruno Falissard, Frédéric Mercier, Hervé Bouaziz, Kamran Samii. Major Complications of Regional Anesthesia in France. Anesthesiology. 2002;97(5):1274–280.
20. Scholten HJ, Pourtaherian A, Mihajlovic N, Korsten HHM, A Bouwman R. Improving needle tip identification during ultrasound-guided procedures in anaesthetic practice. Anaesthesia. 2017;72(7):889–904. https://doi.org/10.1111/anae.13921.
21. Deam RK, Kluger R, Barrington MJ, McCutcheon CA. Investigation of a new echogenic needle for use with ultrasound peripheral nerve blocks. Anaesth Intensive Care. 2007;35(4):582–6. https://doi.org/10.1177/0310057X0703500419.
22. Hebard S, Hocking G. Echogenic technology can improve needle visibility during ultrasound-guided regional anesthesia. Reg Anesth Pain Med. 2011;36:185–9.
23. Henderson M, Dolan J. Challenges, solutions, and advances in ultrasound-guided regional anaesthesia. BJA Educ. 2016;16:mkw026. https://doi.org/10.1093/bjaed/mkw026.
24. Munirama S, McLeod G. Novel applications in ultrasound technology for regional anesthesia. Curr Anesthesiol Rep. 2013;3:230–5. https://doi.org/10.1007/s40140-013-0038-1
25. Kåsine T, Romundstad L, Rosseland LA, et al. The effect of needle tip tracking on procedural time of ultrasound-guided lumbar plexus block: a randomised controlled trial. Anaesthesia. 2020;75(1):72–9. https://doi.org/10.1111/anae.14846.
26. Daoud MI, Alshalalfah AL, Ait Mohamed O, Alazrai R. A hybrid camera- and ultrasound-based approach for needle localization and tracking using a 3D motorized curvilinear ultrasound probe. Med Image Anal. 2018;50:145–66. https://doi.org/10.1016/j.media.2018.09.006.
27. Xia W, Mari JM, West SJ, et al. In-plane ultrasonic needle tracking using a fiber-optic hydrophone. Med Phys. 2015;42(10):5983–91. https://doi.org/10.1118/1.4931418.
28. Rotemberg V, Palmeri M, Rosenzweig S, Grant S, Macleod D, Nightingale K. Acoustic Radiation Force Impulse (ARFI) imaging-based needle visualization. Ultrasonic imaging. 2011;33:1–16.
29. Neal JM, Barrington MJ, Brull R, et al. The second ASRA practice advisory on neurologic complications associated with regional anesthesia and pain medicine: Executive Summary 2015. Reg Anesth Pain Med. 2015;40(5):401–30. https://doi.org/10.1097/AAP.0000000000000286.
30. Gadsden JC, Choi JJ, Lin E, Robinson A. Opening injection pressure consistently detects needle-nerve contact during ultrasound-guided interscalene brachial plexus block. Anesthesiology. 2014;120(5):1246–53. https://doi.org/10.1097/ALN.0000000000000133.
31. Gadsden J, Latmore M, Levine DM, Robinson A. High opening injection pressure is associated with needle-nerve and needle-fascia contact during femoral nerve block. Reg Anesth Pain Med. 2016;41(1):50–5. https://doi.org/10.1097/AAP.0000000000000346.
32. Lin JA, Lu HT. A convenient alternative for monitoring opening pressure during multiple needle redirection. Br J Anaesth. April 2014;112(4):771–2. https://doi.org/10.1093/bja/aeu083.
33. Wahal C, Kumar A, Pyati S. Advances in regional anaesthesia: a review of current practice, newer techniques and outcomes. Indian J Anaesth. 2018;62(2):94–102. https://doi.org/10.4103/ija.IJA_433_17.
34. Lin JA, Blanco R, Shibata Y, Nakamoto T. Advances of techniques in deep regional blocks. Biomed Res Int. 2017;2017:7268308. https://doi.org/10.1155/2017/7268308.

35. Lin JA, Blanco R, Shibata Y, Nakamoto T, Lin KH. Corrigendum to "Advances of Techniques in Deep Regional Blocks". Biomed Res Int. 2018;2018:5151645. https://doi.org/10.1155/2018/5151645. Published 2018 Jul 5.
36. Blanco R. The 'pecs block': a novel technique for providing analgesia after breast surgery. Anaesthesia. 2011;66(9):847–8. https://doi.org/10.1111/j.1365-2044.2011.06838.x.
37. Blanco R, Fajardo M, Parras Maldonado T. Ultrasound description of Pecs II (modified Pecs I): a novel approach to breast surgery. Rev Esp Anestesiol Reanim. 2012;59(9):470–5. https://doi.org/10.1016/j.redar.2012.07.003.
38. Blanco R, Parras T, McDonnell JG, Prats-Galino A. Serratus plane block: a novel ultrasound-guided thoracic wall nerve block. Anaesthesia. 2013 Nov;68(11):1107–13. https://doi.org/10.1111/anae.12344.
39. Nagaraja PS, Ragavendran S, Singh NG, et al. Comparison of continuous thoracic epidural analgesia with bilateral erector spinae plane block for perioperative pain management in cardiac surgery. Ann Card Anaesth. 2018;21(3):323–7. https://doi.org/10.4103/aca.ACA_16_18.
40. Wong WY, Bjørn S, Strid JM, Børglum J, Bendtsen TF. Defining the location of the adductor canal using ultrasound. Reg Anesth Pain Med. 2017;42(2):241–5. https://doi.org/10.1097/AAP.0000000000000539.
41. Conroy PH, Luyet C, McCartney CJ, McHardy PG. Real-time ultrasound-guided spinal anaesthesia: a prospective observational study of a new approach. Anesthesiol Res Pract. 2013;2013:525818. https://doi.org/10.1155/2013/525818.
42. Manohar M, Gupta B, Gupta L. Closed-loop monitoring by anesthesiologists-a comprehensive approach to patient monitoring during anesthesia. Korean J Anesthesiol. 2018;71(5):417–8. https://doi.org/10.4097/kja.d.18.00033.
43. Gholami B, Bailey JM, Haddad WM, Tannenbaum AR. Clinical decision support and closed-loop control for cardiopulmonary management and intensive care unit sedation using expert systems. IEEE Trans Control Syst Technol. 2012;20(5):1343–50. https://doi.org/10.1109/tcst.2011.2162412.
44. Platen PV, Pomprapa A, Lachmann B, et al. The dawn of physiological closed-loop ventilation—a review. Crit Care. 2020;24:121. https://doi.org/10.1186/s13054-020-2810-1
45. Sheahan CG, Mathews DM. Monitoring and delivery of sedation. Br J Anaesth. 2014;113(Suppl 2):ii37–47. https://doi.org/10.1093/bja/aeu378.
46. Uskova A, O'Connor JE. Liposomal bupivacaine for regional anesthesia. Curr Opin Anaesthesiol. 2015;28(5):593–7. https://doi.org/10.1097/ACO.0000000000000240.
47. Pichler L, Poeran J, Zubizarreta N, et al. Liposomal bupivacaine does not reduce inpatient opioid prescription or related complications after knee arthroplasty: a database analysis. Anesthesiology. 2018;129(4):689–99. https://doi.org/10.1097/ALN.0000000000002267.
48. Noviasky J, Pierce DP, Whalen K, Guharoy R, Hildreth K. Bupivacaine liposomal versus bupivacaine: comparative review. Hosp Pharm. 2014;49(6):539–43. https://doi.org/10.1310/hpj4906-539.
49. Liu Y, Zeng Y, Zeng J, et al. The efficacy of liposomal bupivacaine compared with traditional peri-articular injection for pain control following total knee arthroplasty: an updated meta-analysis of randomized controlled trials. BMC Musculoskelet Disord. 2019;20:306.
50. Kirksey MA, Haskins SC, Cheng J, Liu SS. Local anesthetic peripheral nerve block adjuvants for prolongation of analgesia: a systematic qualitative review. PLoS One. 2015;10(9):e0137312. https://doi.org/10.1371/journal.pone.0137312. Published 2015 Sep 10.
51. Marhofer P, Columb M, Hopkins PM, et al. Dexamethasone as an adjuvant for peripheral nerve blockade: a randomised, triple-blinded crossover study in volunteers. Br J Anaesth. 2019;122(4):525–31. https://doi.org/10.1016/j.bja.2019.01.004.
52. Zhang C, Li C, Pirrone M, Sun L, Mi W. Comparison of dexmedetomidine and clonidine as adjuvants to local anesthetics for intrathecal anesthesia: a meta-analysis of randomized controlled trials. J Clin Pharmacol. 2016;56(7):827–34. https://doi.org/10.1002/jcph.666.
53. Vorobeichik L, Brull R, Abdallah FW. Evidence basis for using perineural dexmedetomidine to enhance the quality of brachial plexus nerve blocks: a systematic review and meta-analysis of randomized controlled trials. Br J Anaesth. 2017;118(2):167–81. https://doi.org/10.1093/bja/aew411.

54. Andersen JH, Grevstad U, Siegel H, Dahl JB, Mathiesen O, Jæger P. Does dexmedetomidine have a perineural mechanism of action when used as an adjuvant to ropivacaine?: A paired, blinded, randomized trial in healthy volunteers. Anesthesiology. 2017;126(1):66–73. https://doi.org/10.1097/ALN.0000000000001429.
55. Edwards RM, Currigan DA, Bradbeer S, Mitchell C. Does a catheter over needle system reduce infusate leak in continuous peripheral nerve blockade: a randomised controlled trial. Anaesth Intensive Care. 2018;46(5):468–73. https://doi.org/10.1177/0310057X1804600507.
56. Jordahn ZM, Lyngeraa TS, Grevstad U, et al. Ultrasound guided repositioning of a new suture-method catheter for adductor canal block – a randomized pilot study in healthy volunteers. BMC Anesthesiol. 2018;18:150. https://doi.org/10.1186/s12871-018-0615-4.
57. Finneran JJ IV, Gabriel RA, Swisher MW, et al. Suture catheter for rescue perineural catheter placement when unable to position a conventional through-the-needle catheter: a case report. A Pract. 2019;13(9):338–41. https://doi.org/10.1213/XAA.0000000000001075.
58. Liu S, Wang Y, Yang X et al. Deep Learning in Medical Ultrasound Analysis: A Review. Engineering. 2019;5:261–75.
59. Huang Q, Zhang F, Li X. Machine learning in ultrasound computer-aided diagnostic systems: a survey. Biomed Res Int. 2018;2018:5137904. https://doi.org/10.1155/2018/5137904. Published 2018 Mar 4.
60. Volpato V, Mor-Avi V, Narang A, et al. Automated, machine learning-based, 3D echocardiographic quantification of left ventricular mass. Echocardiography. 2019;36(2):312–9. https://doi.org/10.1111/echo.14234.
61. Medvedofsky D, Mor-Avi V, Byku I, et al. Three-dimensional echocardiographic automated quantification of left heart chamber volumes using an adaptive analytics algorithm: feasibility and impact of image quality in nonselected patients. J Am Soc Echocardiogr. 2017;30(9):879–85. https://doi.org/10.1016/j.echo.2017.05.018.
62. Huang C, Zhou Y, Tan W, et al. Applying deep learning in recognizing the femoral nerve block region on ultrasound images. Ann Transl Med. 2019;7(18):453. https://doi.org/10.21037/atm.2019.08.61.
63. Smistad E, Johansen KF, Iversen DH, Reinertsen I. Highlighting nerves and blood vessels for ultrasound-guided axillary nerve block procedures using neural networks. J Med Imaging (Bellingham). 2018;5(4):044004. https://doi.org/10.1117/1.JMI.5.4.044004.
64. Deserno TM, Oliveira JEE, Grottke O. Regional Anaesthesia Simulator and Assistant (RASimAs): Medical Image Processing Supporting Anaesthesiologists in Training and Performance of Local Blocks. 2015 IEEE 28th International Symposium on Computer-Based Medical Systems, Sao Carlos, 2015, pp. 348–351. https://doi.org/10.1109/CBMS.2015.61.

Safety and Ergonomics of Ultrasound-Guided Regional Anaesthesia

8

Arunangshu Chakraborty and Balakrishnan Ashokka

8.1 Introduction

Regional anaesthesia can become a safer alternative to general anaesthesia when practised meticulously [1–3]. It offers many distinct advantages over general anaesthesia such as

- Patients can remain awake, or minimally sedated, obviating the need for airway management, which is particularly helpful in patients with a difficult airway, obesity-related sleep apnoea and in resource-constrained areas such as the battlefield.
- Nil or minimal need of opioids, and thereby avoiding the burden of addiction, dependence and various side effects of opioids.
- Better pain control.
- It can be administered in patients with uncertain or inadequate fasting status and hence the risk of pulmonary aspiration.

However, it does bring in its own limitations and pitfalls.

The major side effects or complications of regional anaesthesia [4] are

1. *Haematoma: Bruise is noted at the site of injection*

   Particularly in patients with coagulopathies and platelet deficiency. The risk of bleeding and haematoma formation increases in deeper blocks compared to more superficial ones where pressure can be applied to arrest the bleeding. Using ultrasound provides the advantage of real-time imaging of blood vessels thereby

A. Chakraborty
Department of Anaesthesia, CC and Pain, Tata Medical Center, Kolkata, India

B. Ashokka (✉)
National University Health System, Singapore, Singapore

A. Chakraborty (ed.), *Blockmate*, https://doi.org/10.1007/978-981-15-9202-7_8

Table 8.1 Safe dosage limit of local anaesthetic agents

	Plain		With epinephrine	
	Maximum dose			
Local anaesthetic	Per kg BW	Total	Per kg BW	Total
Bupivacaine	2 mg·kg^{-1}	175 mg	3 mg·kg^{-1}	225 mg
Levobupivacaine	2 mg·kg^{-1}	200 mg	3 mg·kg^{-1}	225 mg
Lidocaine	5 mg·kg^{-1}	350 mg	7 mg·kg^{-1}	500 mg
Mepivacaine	5 mg·kg^{-1}	350 mg	7 mg·kg^{-1}	500 mg
Ropivacaine	3 mg·kg^{-1}	200 mg	3 mg·kg^{-1}	250 mg
Prilocaine	6 mg·kg^{-1}	400 mg	8 mg·kg^{-1}	600 mg

decreasing the risk of inadvertent blood vessel injury considerably. A large haematoma can cause pain, fever, pyogenic infection and sequelae including nerve damage due to external compression.

2. *Nerve Injury:*

   The incidence of nerve injury from the block needle is more common in peripheral nerve blocks compared to deeper and neuraxial blocks. On the other hand, the neurological damage in peripheral blocks are usually more transient in nature and rarely cause lasting neuro deficit when compared to neurological damage in a central neuraxial block [5, 6]. The incidence of nerve injury has improved with ultrasound imaging and administration of targeted local anaesthetic in perineural proximity [7–17]

3. *Local Anaesthetic Systemic Toxicity (LAST):*

   LAST can happen if higher than the admissible dosage of LA is used. While calculating dosage, adjustments must be made for extremes of ages, pregnancy, hepatic and renal insufficiency and cardiac disease [18]. One must remember to calculate the dose of the LA with lean body weight. For ease of practice, a total maximum dose is mentioned (Table 8.1) keeping in mind the average height and lean body weight. LAST can happen even within the admissible dosage if rapid vascular absorption happens due to inadvertent intravenous injection or rapid injection in a highly vascular area. The use of ultrasound has reduced the incidence of LAST from 9.8 per 10,000 patients in 2009 to 0.76 in 2018 [10]. It is expected to reduce further as the use of ultrasound for regional anaesthesia as well as regional anaesthesia training programs are gaining momentum worldwide.

   The first step in implementing safety comes in the form of a separate World Health Organisation (WHO) pre-procedural safety checklist for the regional anaesthetic block. Patient identification along with verification of the side and site of the block is of paramount importance (Fig. 8.1).

   The international patient safety goals (IPSG) should be adopted for regional anaesthesia practice as well, which are

   (a) Identify patients correctly (two patient identifiers).
   (b) Improve effective communication.
   (c) Improve the safety of high alert medications.
   (d) Ensure the correct side, correct procedure, correct patient for surgery.
   (e) Reduce the risk of healthcare-associated infections.
   (f) Reduce the risk of patient harm resulting from falls.

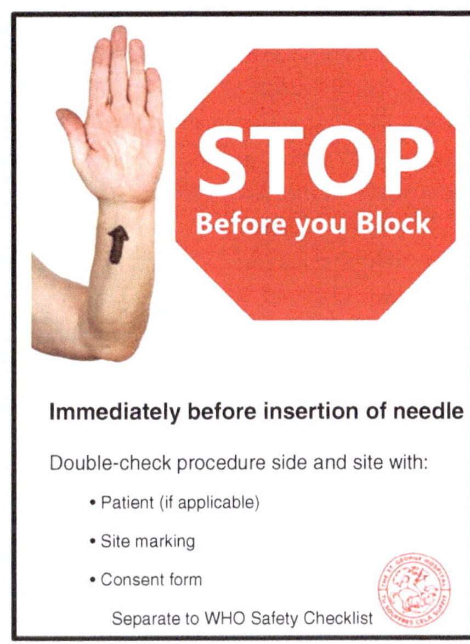

Fig. 8.1 STOP before you block

A focused pre-anaesthesia check-up to find out factors such as smoking, hypertension, polyneuropathy, diabetes, antiplatelet medications, anticoagulation, coagulopathy, thrombocytopenia, etc. could help in the process of decision making as well as understanding the risks involved. Surgery/block should be postponed where possible if the patient is on warfarin or antiplatelet agents. Patients on warfarin need to be switched to heparin or other short acting anticoagulants [19]. Thrombocytopenic patients may need platelet infusion before surgery. The European Society of Anaesthesiologists has published an exhaustive list of time intervals before and after neuraxial puncture or catheter removal [20]. These guidelines are in place to facilitate the safe conduct of regional anaesthesia when the expected pharmacological effects have waned off with the return of normal clotting functions. The practitioner of regional anaesthesia should remember that the evidence suggests that a catheter (neuraxial or PNB) insertion and removal pose a similar risk of bleeding; therefore the same caution should be exercised during removal of a nerve block catheter as inserting it.

8.2 Local Anaesthesia Systemic Toxicity (LAST)

High volume fascial plane block, continuous catheter, multiple blocks in the same patient, tumescent anaesthesia, local infiltration anaesthesia (LIA), etc. are commonly associated with increased risk of LAST [18, 21]. The CNS manifestation is dose dependent. It initially compromises cortical inhibitory pathways by blockade of voltage-gated sodium channels, disrupting inhibitory neuron depolarisation, leading to excitatory clinical features of sensory and visual changes, muscular activation, and subsequent seizure activity. As the plasma concentrations of LA rise, excitatory pathways are affected, producing a depressive phase of neurological toxicity, with loss of consciousness, coma and respiratory arrest.

The cardiovascular manifestations of LAST are potentially fatal. It primarily affects the fast action potentials such as the cardiac rhythm. Normal conduction is disrupted by direct sodium channel blockade, chiefly at the *bundle of His*. By driving the resting membrane potential to a more negative level, action potential propagation is impaired, leading to prolonged PR, QRS, and ST intervals. Re-entrant tachyarrhythmias and bradyarrhythmias ensue, which may be worsened by further potassium channel blockade, prolonging the QT interval. The secondary effects include myocardial dysfunction leading to cardiac arrest and lability of peripheral vascular tone causing profound and refractory hypotension.

The cardiovascular collapse/CNS (CC/CNS) ratio is the ratio of drug dose required to cause catastrophic cardiovascular collapse to the drug dose required to produce seizures. Low CC/CNS ratio means more cardiotoxic agents—because the earlier presentation of CNS features may expedite earlier diagnosis (and treatment) of LAST before cardiovascular collapse ensues.

Ropivacaine and levobupivacaine, for example, have higher CC/CNS ratios than racemic bupivacaine; therefore, it seems logical and safe to preferentially use these drugs when long-acting LAs are desired.

8.3 Clinical Presentation of LAST

- Usually begins within a minute of LA injection but may be delayed, may not always follow the usual sequence. The common sequence of presentations follows:
  - Prodromal symptoms: circum-oral tingling, dizziness, light-headedness, dysarthria, hallucination, delirium. These signs may be masked by dissociative anaesthesia achieved with ketamine, and hence should be used with caution or needs more close monitoring. Seizures and coma.
  - Cardiovascular excitation followed by depression.
  - Malignant arrhythmias and asystole.

8.4 ASRA Guidelines for Management of LAST

1. Prompt and *effective airway management* is crucial to prevent hypoxia and acidosis, which are known to potentiate LAST [22].
2. Seizures should be rapidly halted with *benzodiazepines (BZD)*, If *BZD* is not readily available, small doses of propofol or thiopental are acceptable. The *early use of lipid emulsion for treating seizures is debatable.*

3. *Propofol:* large doses further depress cardiac function, *should be avoided* when there are signs of cardiovascular compromise. If seizures persist despite BZD, *small doses of neuromuscular blocking agents* should be considered to minimize acidosis and hypoxemia.
4. *Cardiac arrest*: ACLS with the following modifications:
   - If epinephrine is used, small initial doses (10–100 μg boluses in the adult) are preferred.
   - Vasopressin is not recommended.
   - Avoid calcium channel blockers and β-adrenergic receptor blockers.
   - If ventricular arrhythmias develop, amiodarone is preferred; lidocaine is not recommended.
5. *Lipid Emulsion Therapy:* Consider lipid rescue therapy at the first signs of LAST, after airway management.

   Dose: 1.5 ml/kg 20% lipid emulsion bolus followed by an infusion of 0.25 ml/kg/min, till at least 10 min after circulatory stability is attained. If circulatory stability is not attained, consider re-bolus and increasing infusion to 0.5 ml/kg/min. About 10 ml/kg lipid emulsion for 30 min is the upper limit for initial dosing.

   Propofol is not a substitute for lipid emulsion.

   Failure to respond to lipid emulsion and vasopressor therapy should prompt the institution of *cardiopulmonary bypass (CPB)*. Because there can be a considerable lag in beginning CPB, it is reasonable to notify the closest facility capable of providing it when cardiovascular compromise is first identified during an episode of LAST.

   Lipid emulsion is a lifesaving drug for the treatment of LAST. All centres where regional anaesthesia is practised should have adequate quantities of it stored. The store should be regularly checked by a formulated inventory management system and a chart kept in a visible area of the operation theatre (e.g. anaesthesia medication trolley) should mention where the nearest lipid unit is kept (Fig. 8.2).

Although LAST happens rarely, when it happens it has a high fatality rate and therefore utmost caution should be taken to avoid it and if detected need to be treated promptly.

A safe maximum dose of local anaesthetics as a guide for preventing the chance of local anaesthetic toxicity is outlined in Table 8.1.

AAGBI Safety Guideline

Management of severe local Anaesthetic Toxicity

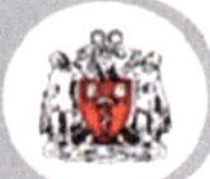

1 Recognition

Signs of severe toxicity:
- Sudden alteration in mental status, severe agitation or loss of consciousness, with or without tonic-clonic convulsions
- Cardiovascular collapse: sinus bradycardla, conduction blocks, asystole and ventricular tachyarrhythmias may all occur
- Local anaesthetic (LA) toxicity may occur some time after an initial injection

2 Immediate management

- Stop injecting the LA
- Call for help
- Maintain the airway and, if necessary, secure it with a tracheal tube
- Give 100% oxygen and ensure adequate lung ventilation (hyperventilation may help by increasing plasma pH in the presence of metabolic acidosis)
- Confirm or establish intravenous access
- Control seizures: give a bezodiazepine, thiopental or propofol in small incremental doses
- Assess cardiovascular status throughout
- Consider drawing blood for analysis, but do not delay definitive treatment to do this

3 Treatment

IN CIRCULATORY ARREST
- Start cardiopuimonary resuscitation (CPR) using standard protocols
- Manage arrhythmias using the same protocols, recognising that arrhythmias may be very refractory to treatment
- Consider the use of cardiopulmonary bypass if available

GIVE INTRAVENOUS LIPID EMULSION
(following the regimen overleaf)
- Continue CPR throughout treatment with lipid emulsion
- Recovery from LA-induced cardiac arrest may take > 1 h
- Propofol is not a suitable substitute for lipid emulsion
- Lidocaine should not be used as an anti-arrhythmic therapy

WITHOUT CIRCULATORY ARREST
Use conventional therapies to treat:
- hypotension,
- bradycardia,
- tachyarrhythmia

CONSIDER INTRAVENOUS LIPID EMULSION
(following the regimen overleaf)
- Propofol is not a suitable substitute for lipid emulsion
- Lidocaine should not be used as an anti-arrhythmic therapy

4 Follow-up

- Arrange safe transfer to a clinical area with approprlate equipment and suitable staff until sustained recovery is achieved
- Exclude pancreatitis by regular clinical review, including daily amylase or lipase assays for two days
- Report cases as follows:
  in the United Kingdom to the National Patient Safety Agency (via www.npsa.nhs.uk)
  in the Republic of Ireland to the irish Medicines Board (via www.imb.ie)

if Lipid has been given, please also report its use to the international registry at www.lipidregistry.org. Details may also be posted at www. lipidrescue.org

Your nearest bag of Lipid Emulsion is kept. ______________________

This guideline is not a standard of medical care. The ultimate judgement with regard to a partioular clinical procedure or treatment plan must be made by the clinician in the light of the clinical data presented and the diagnostic and treatment options available.

Fig. 8.2 AAGBI safety guideline for management of LAST

8.5 Ergonomics of Ultrasound-Guided Regional Anaesthesia

The safety of the conduct of regional anaesthesia lies in how meticulously the process is outlined. All patients who have provided written informed consent are thoroughly assessed for any risks for general anaesthesia and documented before scheduling for a regional anaesthetic. This empowers the team in identifying key considerations when general anaesthesia is to be administered as a rescue technique when regional anaesthetics fail or is patchy or for management of untoward events requiring cardiopulmonary resuscitation.

8.5.1 Location: Place of Conduct

The administration of regional anaesthetic should be permitted only in patient care locations that have the capacity to support oxygenation and safe management of circulation. There are three common practice locations for regional anaesthetic administration: in theatre/on table, induction or ante-room and designated regional anaesthetic block areas (RABA). Administration in operation theatres and RABA are usually considered safe as both locations are generally equipped with qualified regional anaesthesia experts who can provide continued care for the patients before and after the administration of local anaesthetic and sedation. Induction or ante-room administration of RA though might be practiced for enhancing theatre efficiency, is often fraught with the concerns of either one of the patients in the operating theatre or ante-room being at risk from lapse in attention from the attending anaesthesiologist. The presence of time pressure and constant auditory inputs from the patient emergence cues from inside the operating room could be a distraction to the proceduralist. Ante-room procedures are performed only when there is a committed and qualified healthcare professional designated to be present with the patient before and after the procedure. They should be capable of recognising and escalating the occurrence of cardiorespiratory compromise and other post-procedural complications.

Optimising the user comfort during the administration of RA is important. This will include the use of noise/distraction limited place, optimum height of procedure area, the placement of the machine, patient and proceduralist in a line, the technique, patient position, direction of needling (towards or away from proceduralist), type of probe, way the probe is held, support personnel and near point adjustment (Table 8.2).

Table 8.2 Key points of USRA ergonomics

Feature	Conduct	Additional points
Table/bed height	Adjust to umbilical height of proceduralist	Reduces stooping, shoulder, and back strain
Near point	Optimally achieved between 30 and 60 cm	Avoids parallax error, having a picture and not missing needle path
Patient position	Patient in best position of comfort, and optimum level of table adjustment	Minimises probe contact with undesired surface, achieves best USG view
Needle view on USG	In plane versus out of plane	In plane is suitable for novices; out of plane use requires advanced understanding of anatomical structures
Needle direction	Towards the proceduralist versus away from the proceduralist	Common mode of administration is away from the proceduralist, needling towards requires advanced needle control and understanding of three-dimensional needle progress
Needle holding	Pencil holding technique	Provides optimum needle pressure, feel of tissues resistance, avoids injury, and feel of give when crossing tissue planes
Three point alignment (3 P) (Fig. 8.3)	Proceduralist, probe, picture	All three in a straight line alignment; avoids undue movements, reduces vascular and nerve injury

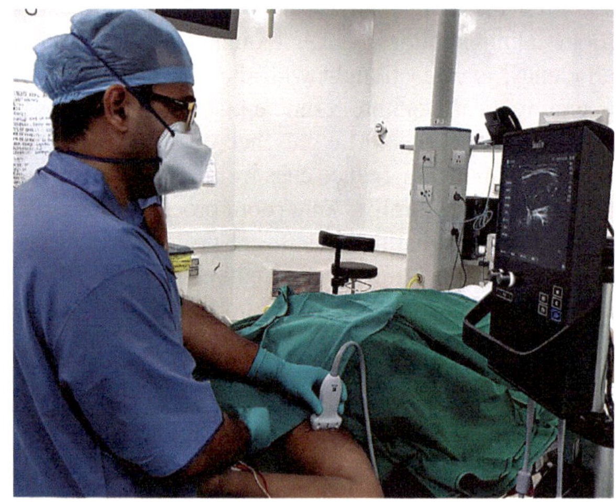

Fig. 8.3 Optimal positioning for ultrasound guided nerve bloack placements, the table height is adjusted to the waist level. The proceduralist, the probe and the US monitor (picture)—all three 'P's are aligned in a straight line

An operating theatre regional anaesthetic set up should facilitate optimal ergonomics (Fig. 8.4). The regional anaesthesia specialist is supported by theatre technician for achieving optimal patient positioning, operating table conditions. Anaesthesia nurse/assistant provides technical support equipment, drugs and consumables, enhances sterile practice advisories, and provides patient monitoring and has resuscitation capabilities when required. Regional anaesthetic equipment should be placed in front of the proceduralist and regional anaesthetic trolley positioned on the side of the dominant hand of the proceduralist. This provides opportunity for

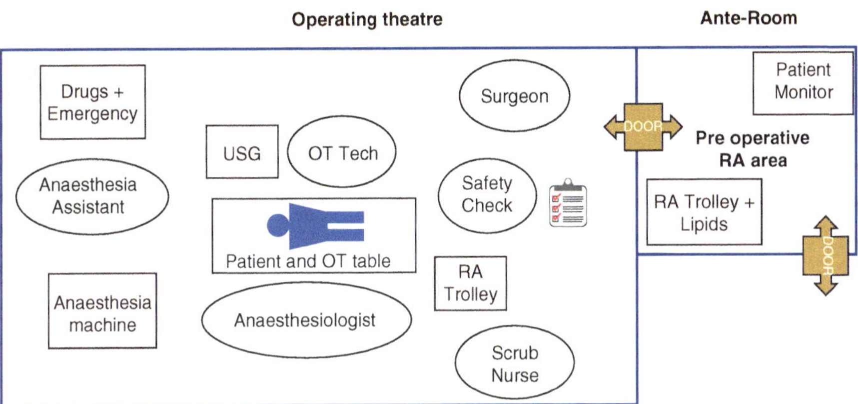

Fig. 8.4 The schematic for operating theatres and ante-room anaesthetic administrations with an outline for the theatre personnel, equipment and resuscitation facilities

monitoring patient all through the procedure, enabling optimum visualisation of the relevant structures in anatomical orientation along the axis of sonography performed. Equipment and drugs for resuscitation and additional personnel such as the surgeon and theatre scrub nurse must be available within the theatre. Performing the immediate pre-procedural safety checklist and operating site localisation by participation from the conscious patient, before sedation is commenced, enhances the overall safety, minimises wrong-site procedures and enhances patient satisfaction.

8.5.2 Role of Simulation

Simulation in its full spectrum helps in enhancing the safety of the conduct of regional anaesthetic (Table 8.3). Part task simulations are useful in enhancing technical finesse by enhancing deliberate practice to achieve proficiency in regional anaesthesia techniques such as probe orientations, needle trajectory and its steady placement within tissues. Large jelly-filled spine models are known to provide three-dimensional orientation to depth, needle path and hand–eye coordination [23]. Cadaveric and live animal model simulations are known to enhance the actual tissue feedback and planning for these formats of simulations can be laborious with a fully maintained wet lab facility. Intermediate fidelity/technology simulations can be practiced for enhancing drill-based compliance to set protocols for resuscitations such as ACLS for any cardiopulmonary collapse, or even be simulated through simple 'call out' card-based role-playing exercises with stand-alone virtual simulated tablet screens. Full-scale simulations with multidisciplinary team simulations are recommended every 6months to facilitate team training and interpersonal communications [24]. This enhances the safety in learning from previous sentinel events, reiterating the root cause analysis, the proposed practice advisories that are in line with regional and global standards [25].

Table 8.3 Simulations and role for enhancing regional anesthesia safety

Type of simulation	Domain	Specific outcomes	Features
Part task training	Psychomotor	Enhanced needling techniques, needle visualisations hand–eye coordination	Jelly block, agar or cellulose filled small segments
Cadaveric training	Psychomotor Cognitive	Tissue plane haptic feedback, anatomical tissue negotiations	Needs preservation and thawing; expensive, rarity to get cadavers
Live tissues training (animals)	Psychomotor Cognitive Emotive	Real-time tissues plane feedback with warmth and vascular structure pulsatality and respiratory excursions	Performed in conjunction with live workshops with other specialties like surgery; needs regulatory clearance
Intermediate fidelity trainers	Critical thinking skills; psychomotor resus skills	Time-based drills for protocol-based management; use of cognitive aids for safe management	Enhances team confidence in rescue and emergency skills; can be used for assessments
Full-scale simulations	Leadership skills, soft skills	Scenario-based team outcomes; multiprofessional participations and collective decision making	Costly mannequins, faculty and resource intensive

Regional anaesthetics tend to be preferred in patients who have multiple comorbidities with limited cardiopulmonary reserves. Provision of regional anaesthetic should be considered with the similar precautions as for a general anaesthetic and not be discounted to be 'local anaesthesia with sedation'. The safety lies in planning, anticipation of crisis, preparation of the theatre, equipment, drugs and personnel to respond in a timely and coordinated manner.

References

1. Marhofer P. Safe performance of peripheral regional anaesthesia: the significance of ultrasound guidance. Anaesthesia. 2017;72:427–38.
2. Koscielniak-Nielsen ZJ. Ultrasound guided peripheral nerve blocks: what are the benefits? Acta Anaesthesiol Scand. 2008;52:727–37.
3. Halsted WS. Practical comments on the use and abuse of cocaine. N Y Med J. 1885;42:294–5.
4. Barrington MJ, Watts SA, Gledhill SR, Thomas RD, Said SA, Snyder GL, Tay VS, Jamrozik K. Preliminary results of the Australasian Regional Anaesthesia Collaboration: a prospective audit of more than 7000 peripheral nerve and plexus blocks for neurologic and other complications. Reg Anesth Pain Med. 2009 Oct 1;34(6):534–41.
5. Bigeleisen PE. Nerve puncture and apparent intraneural injection during ultrasound-guided axillary block does not invariably result in neurologic injury. Anesthesiology. 2006;105:779–83.
6. Bigeleisen PE, Moayeri N, Groen GJ. Extraneural versus intraneural stimulation thresholds during ultrasound guided supraclavicular block. Anesthesiology. 2009;110:1235–43.
7. Sermeus LA, Sala-Blanch X, McDonnell JG, et al. Ultrasound-guided approach to nerves (direct vs. tangential) and the incidence of intraneural injection: a cadaveric study. Anaesthesia. 2017;72:461–9.

8. Abrahams MS, Aziz MF, Fu RF, Horn J. Ultrasound guidance compared with electrical neurostimulation for peripheral nerve block: a systematic review and meta-analysis of randomized controlled trials. Br J Anaesth. 2009;102:408–17.
9. Lewis SR, Price A, Walker KJ, McGrattan K, Smith AF. Ultrasound guidance for upper and lower limb blocks. Cochrane Database Syst Rev. 2015;11:CD006459.
10. Munirama S, McLeod G. A systematic review and meta-analysis of ultrasound versus electrical stimulation for peripheral nerve location and blockade. Anaesthesia. 2015;70:1084–91.
11. Chandra A, Eisma R, Felts P, Munirama S, McLeod G. The feasibility of microultrasound as a tool to image peripheral nerves. Anaesthesia. 2017;72:190–6.
12. Robards C, Hadzic A, Somasundaram L, et al. Intraneural injection with low current stimulation during popliteal sciatic nerve block. Anesth Analg. 2009;109:673–7.
13. Chan VWS, Brull R, McCartney CJL, Xu D, Abbas S, Shannon P. An ultrasonographic and histological study of intraneural injection and electrical stimulation in pigs. Anesth Analg. 2007;04:1281–4.
14. Kirchmair L, Strohle M, Loscher WN, Kreutziger J, Voelckel WG, Lirk P. Neurophysiological effects of needle trauma and intraneural injection in a porcine model: a pilot study. Acta Anaesthesiol Scand. 2016;60:393–9.
15. Liguori GA. Complications of regional anesthesia: nerve injury and peripheral neural blockade. J Neurosurg Anesthesiol. 2004;16:84–6.
16. Brull R, Hadzic A, Reina MA, Barrington MJ. Pathophysiology and etiology of nerve injury following peripheral nerve blockade. Reg Anesth Pain Med. 2015;40:479–90.
17. Brull R, McCartney CJL, Chan VWS, ElBeheiry H. Neurological complications after regional anesthesia: contemporary estimates of risk. Anesth Analg. 2007;104:965–74.
18. Walker BJ, Long JB, Sathyamoorthy M, Birstler J, Wolf C, Bosenberg AT, Flack SH, Krane EJ, Sethna NF, Suresh S, Taenzer AH. Complications in pediatric regional anesthesia. An analysis of more than 100,000 blocks from the pediatric regional anesthesia network. Anesthesiology. 2018 Oct 1;129(4):721–32.
19. Horlocker TT, Vandermeuelen E, Kopp SL, Gogarten W, Leffert LR, Benzon HT. Regional Anesthesia in the Patient Receiving Antithrombotic or Thrombolytic Therapy: American Society of Regional Anesthesia and Pain Medicine Evidence-Based Guidelines (Fourth Edition) [published correction appears in Reg Anesth Pain Med. 2018 Jul;43(5):566. Vandermeuelen, Erik [corrected to Vandermeulen, Erik]]. Reg Anesth Pain Med. 2018;43(3):263–309. https://doi.org/10.1097/AAP.0000000000000763.
20. Gogarten W, Vandermeulen E, van Aken H, Kozek S, Llau JV, Samama CM. Regional anaesthesia and antithrombotic agents: recommendations of the European Society of Anaesthesiology. Eur J Anaesthesiol. 2010;27:999–1015.
21. Sites BD, et al. Incidence of local anesthetic systemic toxicity and postoperative neurologic symptoms associated with 12,668 ultrasound-guided nerve blocks: an analysis from a prospective clinical registry. Reg Anesth Pain Med. 2012;37(5):478–82.
22. Rubin DS, Matsumoto MM, Weinberg G, et al. Local anesthetic systemic toxicity in total joint arthroplasty: incidence and risk factors in the United States from the National Inpatient Sample 1998–2013. Reg Anesth Pain Med. 2018;43:131–7.
23. Karmakar MK, Ki Jinn Chin KJ. Spinal sonography and applications of ultrasound for central neuraxial blocks. NYSORA. https://www.nysora.com/techniques/neuraxial-and-perineuraxial-techniques/spinal-sonography-and-applications-of-ultrasound-for-central-neuraxial-blocks/. Accessed 10 Jul 2020.
24. Ashokka B, Dong C, Law LS, Liaw SY, Chen FG, Samarasekera DD. A BEME systematic review of teaching interventions to equip medical students and residents in early recognition and prompt escalation of acute clinical deteriorations: BEME Guide No. 62. Medical Teacher. 2020;1–14. Advance online publication. https://doi.org/10.1080/0142159X.2020.1763286.
25. American Society of Regional Anesthesia and Pain Medicine (ASRA): Safety and guidelines. https://www.asra.com/page/1462/safety-and-guidelines. Accessed 10 Jul 2020.